THE WILDATARIAN DIET

LIVING AS NATURE INTENDED

A customized nutritional approach
For optimal health, energy, and vitality

ISBN-13: 978-0-692-06744-4 (ebook)
ISBN-13: 978-0-692-06743-7 (print)

Book design and recipe photography by Lindsay Benson Garrett, Copper Note
Author photo by Jaime Sanchez
Credits: Some graphics courtesy of Vecteezy, Pexels, Depositphotos, and iStock. All copyrights belong to their respective owners.

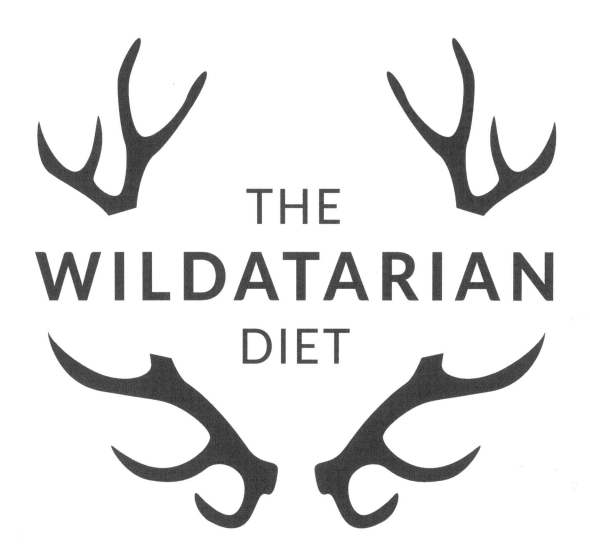

THE
WILDATARIAN
DIET

LIVING AS NATURE INTENDED

*A customized nutritional approach
for optimal health, energy, and vitality*

BY TERI COCHRANE
NUTRITIONAL COUNSELOR & INTEGRATIVE PRACTITIONER, CCP

This book is dedicated to my children, William and Madeleine.
They are the inspiration behind my work and my practice.
They are my greatest teachers.

To my mother, who instilled in me a love of family.

To my father, who taught me to never stop learning.

CONTENTS

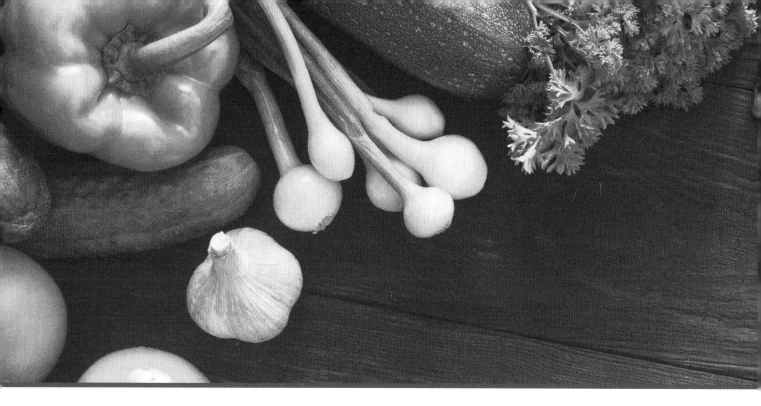

WILDATARIAN™ | NOUN:

1. *A dietary and lifestyle regimen consisting of the consumption of generally wild-caught, wild-fed, and sustainable animal and plant-based proteins that have not been industrially raised, processed, genetically modified, hormonally or bacterially supplemented, or in any way divergent from their whole, natural form. This includes wild game meats and fowl, such as bison, venison, elk, goat, lamb, pheasant, and quail; wild-caught fish and shellfish; ancient, organic, non-chemically altered or treated grains; organic, non-mycotoxic legumes, nuts, seeds, and produce; and organic, generally grass-fed, non-hormonally treated dairy products. This is a lifestyle that fosters a practice of abundance, positivity, and intentional living. This is a lifestyle that affirms a greater connection with community and planet. It is a commitment to personal engagement. It is a pledge to be proactive, and to seek, commit to, and live a life of abundance as nature intended.*

2. *One who consumes wild and sustainable proteins, grains, legumes, nuts, seeds, and produce for vibrant, total-body health on a molecular level.*

WILDATARIAN | ADJECTIVE

1. *A way of eating and living that encompasses **Wildatarian** principles.*

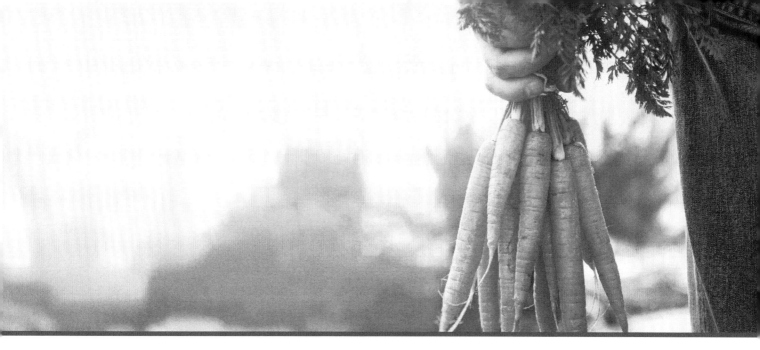

PREFACE

If my life's journey has taught me one thing, it is that the student may one day become the teacher. I have dedicated the last eighteen years of my life to seeking health solutions—first within my own family and later with clients in my private practice.

I did not set out to become a nutritional counselor or an integrative practitioner. I followed a typical path: I went to college and became a banker, then bankruptcy specialist, then portfolio services director at Freddie Mac, where I was tasked with overseeing the health of multifamily assets.

But life had something else in store for me. My son's illness at a young age forced me to start looking at lifestyle and nutrition. And once I got started, I could not stop. My analytical mind made connections and compelled me to continue studying. I was a financial risk manager, and I soon became a risk manager for my son's health.

MY FAMILY'S STORY

My son, now twenty-three, spent his early life struggling with life-threatening asthma, bleeding eczema, recurrent strep infections, and a failure to thrive. He was born six weeks premature.

I was working full time in real estate finance, and because I did not understand the benefits of breast milk at the time I stopped nursing when he was three months old.

Although he had been born prematurely, the first eighteen months of his life were fortunately uneventful. I thought I was feeding him healthfully by providing formula, homemade soups, and purees made with vegetables and meats. He appeared to be a happy, healthy baby. He was placed appropriately on the growth charts, and was rarely sick. At eighteen months, everything changed. I started regularly feeding him peanut butter and jelly sandwiches, orange juice, and chicken nuggets. Concurrently, he received his eighteen-month vaccinations. These two factors formed the perfect storm for autoimmune symptomatology to present in his body. He developed a host of conditions, including severe bleeding eczema on his face and body, severe asthma symptoms, and allergic shiners (dark circles under the eyes, which can indicate food sensitivities). His skin tone was altered as well.

And so it began—from eighteen months until the age of ten, my son's life changed dramatically. In an effort to manage his life-threatening asthma, a schedule of oral and inhaled steroids and bronchodilators became his regular, recurring treatment. At his three-year-old "well check" with our pediatrician, we learned his bone density was that of a nineteen-month-old because of the repeated steroid use. He had fallen off the growth chart, and I was told not to expect him to grow past five-feet, four inches tall ... but to prepare for brain seizures. By age five, my son was regularly in the hospital.

Long-term use of steroids can suppress adrenal function (our anti-inflammatory glands), lead to adrenal fatigue, contribute to candida and other fungal infections in the body, lower bone density, and promote insulin and glucose imbalance. My son was the victim of the deleterious effects of medications that were needed to save his life. During his first year in school, he contracted strep eleven times. And so it went—a cycle of multiple illnesses, countless prescriptions, and failure to thrive.

Looking for more answers, I turned to a doctor trained in holistic methods. Tests (including saliva, stool, and blood) showed my son was unable to properly process wheat (a poorly digestible protein), dairy (mucus producing food, which exacerbates asthma), peanuts and corn, which contain mycotoxins (fungi metabolites that can trigger mold toxicity and contribute to candida, asthma, and eczema), and orange juice (sugar and acid, which feed eczema, candida, and mold). I immediately removed these offending foods from his diet and then saw some symptom improvement. The road to full recovery would take much longer, as his immune system was weakened by a combination of bad food, vaccines, pathogens, and medications. I now call this *systemic reactivity*, which means his entire body became indiscriminately reactive to foods and the environment, making him very sick. This is when I left my twenty-year corporate career to find a solution to his health crisis.

With the body of knowledge I have accumulated over the last eighteen years, I now can explain what happened to my son. His life experiences had made him susceptible to various pathogens and indigestible large proteins. Understanding his genetic profile also shed light on the progression of his illness. Both my son and my daughter share three genetic polymorphisms with me. **Polymorphism** is a term used in genetics to describe multiple forms of a single gene that exist in an individual or among a group of individuals. In some cases, a polymorphism can manifest in negative ways. These polymorphisms were:

- **METHYLATION.** According to pharmacist Suzy Cohen, "Methylation is the process of taking a single carbon and three hydrogens, known as a methyl group, and applying it to many critical functions in your body such as: thinking, repairing DNA, turning on and off genes, fighting infections, and getting rid of environmental toxins to name a few." This can translate to being less likely to digest protein, as the body lacks methyl donors that support the production of hydrochloric acid necessary for digestion of proteins and for the breakdown of pathogens.
- **SULFATION.** Sulfation is an important pathway of metabolism for a range of internal compounds, including steroid hormones, bile acids, neurotransmitters, and small peptides. Impaired sulfation is linked to asthma and eczema.
- **CYTOCHROME P450 GENE FAMILY.** This refers to a group of enzymes involved in drug metabolism and found in high levels in the liver. These enzymes change many drugs, including anticancer drugs, into less toxic forms that are easier for the body to excrete. Someone with polymorphisms in this gene family may be less likely to process drugs, substances, and toxins.

My son had a trifecta of vulnerable genes. The steroids further depleted adrenal function and allowed the pathogens of strep, candida, and mold to flourish in his body. His digestive system and gut biome[1] kept taking hit after hit.

It took years of a clean diet and supportive supplements to rebalance his system, but he is now a healthy, happy young man who no longer suffers from asthma or eczema. He was my first and, at the time, most important client. As I researched, studied, and learned, he continued to heal. He graduated from the University of Virginia in the spring of 2017, and was a five-foot, eleven-inch tall Junior Olympic gold medalist in karate, a multi-sport athlete, and a gifted musician and scholar.

My next big step in learning started years later when my daughter became septic after a botched wisdom-tooth extraction at age fifteen. It was so severe that she spent several days in the hospital. The lifesaving IV antibiotic clindamycin likely shifted her gut biome, allowing candida to overgrow, which caused a host of food sensitivities. Nine months later, while spending the summer at a ballet conservatory she was incorrectly dispensed a supplement over several weeks, causing her liver to become toxic. This otherwise healthy, beautiful, and brilliant young woman once again became very sick. She stopped mensing and lost the ability to properly regulate her body temperature. Her insulin skyrocketed, she started losing hair, and experienced repeated episodes of fainting. Eventually, her face became puffy, and her blood pressure dropped to dangerously low levels. Because her digestion and liver were so compromised, she contracted E. coli from tainted food a few months later. Then as she entered senior year in high school and was on a pre-professional ballet track, she was forced to give up dancing. All her other health challenges, including osteomyelitis, a serious condition caused by Staphylococcus aureus, a form of staph that infects the bone, were taxing her once-strong body. Her blood work also showed dangerous levels of biotoxins (harmful molds and toxins in her body).

We consulted with multiple mainstream and integrative doctors across the country, and not one could resolve her symptoms. My mission to understand the trajectory of her declining health allowed me to launch the next phase of my practice—incorporating how the body expresses genes—into my thinking. One of my staff members, who is a trained scientist with a past job as a researcher at the National Institutes of Health, dove into genetics. She found scientific studies that supported what I was seeing with my daughter and with other clients in my practice.

---

1   The gut biome is a collection of microorganisms that live in our intestinal tract, made up of communities of symbiotic, commensal, and pathogenic bacteria, fungi, and viruses that create a sort of mini-ecosystem. When this system becomes disrupted, a disease state can follow.

For my daughter, a perfect storm of pathogens and liver toxicity shifted the expression in her genes and made her less able to digest proteins and fats. An interplay between bacterial pathogens and the Epstein-Barr virus (EBV), the virus that triggers mononucleosis, combined to damage her digestive tract, tax her immune system, and cause systemic inflammation.

In addition, her body was regularly producing excess epinephrine (aka adrenaline, one of the stress hormones) because of her rigorous ballet training schedule. This excess epinephrine caused a breach in her intestinal barrier, further weakening her immune system. (Epinephrine has been shown clinically to contribute to the rise of pathogenic bacteria in the gut.) Her immune system was already taxed from the pathogens of EBV, candida, staph, and E. coli. In addition, the excess epinephrine was further congesting an already delicate liver, making it harder for her body to process fats and other fat-soluble molecules such as estrogen, insulin, thyroid, and pituitary hormones.

This was her perfect storm. Because of the candida and bacterial infections which feed on sugar and carbohydrates, she was eating a high-protein, non-**Wildatarian**, low-carb diet. Such foods are often recommended for those with these infections. The amyloids from the non-wild meats and poultry were further fortifying the pathogens we were trying to kill. Amyloids will be further defined later in the book, but essentially they are aggregates of less-digestible proteins that contribute to feeding pathogens. Her path to health started when we placed her on a low-fat, **Wildatarian** food plan. She is now back to good health and thriving at a top university, studying international policy, environmental science, and ballet.

Both of my children recovered from life-threatening illnesses when I discerned the root cause of their imbalance and when they changed the way they ate to support their unique genetic blueprint.

> **Wildatarianism** is the foundational element of my private practice protocol. For people who cannot see me or have less complex health concerns, I developed the **Wildatarian** consumer model to allow them to reach their physical and emotional potential. The method relies on truthful answers to a set of questions packaged into a quiz, which can be taken online. The goal of the quiz is to determine which of the four **Wildatarian** types a person falls into—types designed around the malabsorption of the **Wildatarian** Big Three: protein, fat, and sulfur.

My approach to health is creating a buzz around the holistic health world. The clients I see tend to come to me as a last resort after seeing multiple other practitioners at elite institutions across the United States. I have helped rebalance their bodies and facilitated their unique and highest level of health. My practice illuminates certain fallacies behind main-stream dietary advice being dispensed today—advice such as *kale is the king of vegetables, grains are the root of all evil,* or *follow a ketogenic diet.* Popular diets that remove entire food groups don't allow our bodies to live up to their full potential; I begin from the principle that no diet works for everyone.

FINDING THE *TRU OF YOU*™

This book is about finding the *Tru of You.* The **Wildatarian** approach and lifestyle help you find your individual truth—to optimize health, manage stress, and realize the physical, emotional, and spiritual balance that nature intended. This is the genesis of a miraculous transformation that helps sustain a vibrant, healthy you.

This book is my love letter to a more common-sense and natural approach to food and life. In it, I encourage you to eat mindfully and celebrate the whole nutrition Mother Nature provides. By following your bio-individual **Wildatarian** approach, you will support a healthy gut biome, avoid taxing your system with foods that may negatively affect the expression of genes, and foster a lifestyle of intentional and balanced living. These tenets have proven—not only with my children, but with the thousands of clients I have seen for over a decade—that nothing is impossible to rebalance, heal, and strengthen.

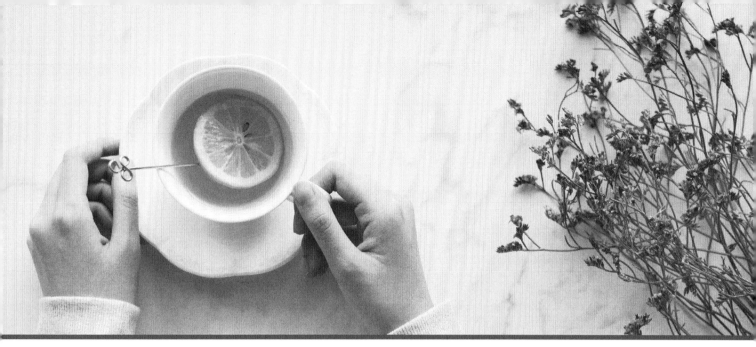

INTRODUCTION

Hippocrates wrote, "*Let food be thy medicine*," and those words speak an eternal truth. This book provides a groundbreaking look into how imbalance may manifest in your body as the result of your diet, nutritional and supplemental choices, your unique genetics, and your stress response.

Your body is a brilliant machine that works around the clock, managing countless processes to maintain homeostasis and health. When toxic and emotional burdens reach a tipping point, the body's ability to maintain balance is lost.

Because we each have a unique genetic blueprint, there is no one healthy food for *everyone*. As one of my nutritional counselors espouses, *genes are tendency, not destiny*. We have learned that we can use our genetic blueprint as a map to teach us how to navigate our innate predispositions and work with them to heal from disease and optimize health. This is central to the **Wildatarian** approach, and this book and the online quiz provide your unique map to determine your **Wildatarian** type.

Stress is a monstrous catalyst for altering gene expression. Negative consequences may occur if particular genes are expressed or "turned on." Certain genes can manifest as inabilities to process particular foods, while others can reduce our capacity to manage or combat viruses, bacteria, and other pathogens. These impairments can, in turn, lead to intolerances, allergies, and ailments that riddle us with poor health and a diminished vitality.

A healthy gut biome encompasses microorganisms that live in our intestinal tract and is made up of communities of symbiotic, commensal, and pathogenic bacteria, fungi, and viruses that create a type of a mini- ecosystem. By following the Standard American Diet, we are eating food treated with pesticides, supplemental hormones, antibiotics, artificial colors, and sugars. This diet fuels an imbalance in pathogens such as viruses, yeasts and bacteria, which then impacts our bodies' immune function. The Standard American Lifestyle, with its unending stressors, is disrupting the integrity of our gut microbiome and further fueling these pathogens.

Together, the Standard American Diet and our stress-filled lives (collectively termed as the Standard American Lifestyle) are contributing to an inflammatory cascade in our bodies, leading to autoimmunity and disease.

Autoimmune conditions are increasing at an alarming rate. Autoimmunity is defined as a misdirected immune response where the body attacks its own cells. A generation ago, autoimmunity was rare. Now, we are experiencing conditions such as Crohn's disease, Type 1 diabetes, endocrine imbalances, mental health disorders, rheumatoid arthritis, and autoimmune thyroid disease at exponentially increasing levels. Many more autoimmune conditions are either under-recognized or unaddressed. Researchers estimate that one in nine of us is affected by autoimmunity.

THE BIG THREE OF MALABSORPTION: PROTEIN, FAT, AND SULFUR

In more than ten years of extensive research and clinical outcomes, I have found that the malabsorption of protein, fat, and sulfur has become one of the biggest contributors to America's collective current state of imbalance. I refer to these variables as The Big Three.

My research shows that The Big Three can impact genetic expression, alter detoxification pathways, and increase pathogenicity in our bodies. Our food supply and our lifestyles put a toxic burden on our bodies, which disrupts absorption and assimilation of proteins, fats, and sulfur, tampering with how our genes are expressed.

UNDERSTANDING PROTEIN: ABNORMAL PROTEINS AND AMYLOIDS

Proteins are molecules composed of one or more chains of amino acids in a specific order; they serve as building blocks in our body. They are required for the structure, function, and regulation of the body's cells, tissues, and organs. We consume protein in our diet from a variety of sources. Our bodies know how to break these proteins down into amino acids to be used for many of its critical functions. We must recognize the beauty and craftsmanship through which nature has designed its many biological processes, for we may see how the naturally occurring proteins found in consumable animal meat have historically served as repairing and anti-inflammatory agents within our bodies. However, the rise of the modern meat production industry, with its crowded spaces, supplemental hormones, antibiotics, and herbicides and pesticides, have significantly modified not only the quality of conventional meat products but also their composition on a molecular level.

Through research, we have seen how the proteins within conventionally produced meat have the ability to become truncated and misfolded into structures known as amyloids, which may not be easily assimilated by the body. This alteration in structure may have deleterious effects on the body's ability to break down and absorb these proteins, which are essential to creating amino acids for the structure of the body and as building blocks for enzymes, antibodies, and hormones. When we consume conventional meat containing abnormal proteins, the human body may not recognize their fragmented and altered structure, and may be unable to break them down as intended. New research shows that amyloids are linked to innumerable chronic diseases—including Type 1 diabetes, Alzheimer's, Parkinson's, and autoimmune disease.

The discovery of amyloids and their significance in contributing to disease states has revolutionized my approach to looking at the body and health. The **Wildatarian** diet aims to reduce dietary amyloids and shift toward protein structures that are not only nourishing but also healing. For despite what nature has intended, the food we eat has gone from nourishing to devastating.

Studies have found that dietary amyloids occur in commercial beef and chicken but are likely found in most inflamed animals—animals burdened by internal infections, antibiotics, and foods that are indigestible for them.

UNDERSTANDING FAT: STRESS RESPONSE AND BODY BURDEN

Fat, along with protein and carbohydrates, is a macronutrient. Fat is the major unit of stored energy in the body. Most of the stored fat in our bodies exists in a form called triglycerides, which are three individual fatty acids connected by another molecule, glycerol. Approximately 60 percent of brain matter is made up of fats. Therefore, proper fat metabolism and absorption is critical to brain and cognitive function.

Consuming a diet high in fat can cause genetically vulnerable people to become fat malabsorbed—creating a state of not being able to properly metabolize fats, which can clog their livers and intoxicate their systems. Our Standard American Lifestyle, with its associated high and relentless stress levels, causes a constant secretion of epinephrine—a fat-based hormone that can slow the processing of fats by the body and actually wreak havoc on the integrity of our digestive system and immune function. The stress response can disrupt our ability to manage hormones that are fat soluble, further exacerbating the fat malabsorption. When the body cannot break down and assimilate fat, the benefits of healthy constituents such as omega-3s and monounsaturated fatty acids are less available to us. In fact, in this state we may increase our body burden and promote dysfunction such as gut permeability, clogged liver, impaired hormone metabolism, and acne.

The **Wildatarian** diet can help you figure out how much dietary fat is appropriate for you—something that is extremely important, especially with the rising popularity of high-fat diets.

UNDERSTANDING SULFUR: A POTENTIAL TOXIC BURDEN

Sulfur is a compound that is found in many foods, medications, and supplements. It has to be metabolized by our body's detoxification pathways. One unspoken paradox of current dietary advice is that healthy, sulfur-rich foods, such as kale and broccoli, may be contributing to diseases such as Crohn's, ulcerative colitis, arthritis, and even mental health conditions.

Cruciferous vegetables, onions, garlic, and other similar foods are the darlings of most dietary advice in the market today. Smoothies and green juices often feature these foods, and the public is encouraged to consume as many of them as possible. For some individuals, these foods are difficult to digest at best, and harmful at worst.

Many things in our environment may impact sulfur metabolism. A big contributor is gluten, a large plant-based protein found in the grains of wheat, rye, barley, spelt, and kamut. Glyphosate, the herbicide sprayed on our crops, is also contributing to this disruption. Mycotoxins, found in our largest crops of corn, soy, peanuts, and certain other legumes, can also affect sulfur processing. When this pathway is disrupted, we feel sick, stressed, and tired and are more susceptible to certain mental health and autoimmune disorders such as depression and ulcerative colitis.

The **Wildatarian** diet helps you determine if you are vulnerable to the sulfur burden and when you should be careful with these compounds.

RESTORING THE BODY WITH CLEAN AND HEALTHY EATING

Every day in our practice, we work with a variety of individuals who have a range of health conditions. These individuals have benefited from eating a bio-individual diet—which sometimes means omitting trendy "health" foods—and thereby experiencing the positive results that years of eating traditionally accepted "healthy" foods did not provide.

I have learned that the gut biome, with its natural barrier function, and the immune system thrive when you do the following:

- Minimize or eliminate foods that cannot be easily assimilated by the body based on your genetic blueprint and current state of health
- Minimize or eliminate offending foods, such as those containing amyloids, gluten, and glyphosates.
- Consume easily digestible forms of protein, certain gluten-free grains, nuts, seeds,

legumes, and vegetables that are low in mycotoxins, mold, and glyphosates.

- Focus on the fats that your body can assimilate and use.
- Switch to natural sugars that do not tax your blood sugar regulation and stress response.

YOUR WILDATARIAN TYPE

Because each one of us is distinctive, I have established four major **Wildatarian** types based on each individual's unique genetic blueprint and current health status. They are:

- **W–TYPE Wildatarian™ Basic**

  Eliminates gluten and beef, pork/ham, chicken, and turkey
- **WS–TYPE Wildatarian™ (Low-Sulfur)**

  Eliminates gluten, beef, pork/ham, chicken, and turkey, and foods rich in dietary sulfur, such as egg yolks, some shellfish, garlic, and cruciferous vegetables
- **WF–TYPE Wildatarian™ (Low-Fat)**

  Eliminates gluten, beef, pork/ham, chicken, and turkey, and foods with a higher fat content or those containing harder-to-digest fats
- **WFS–TYPE Wildatarian™ (Low-Fat and Low-Sulfur)**

  Eliminates gluten, beef, pork/ham, chicken, and turkey, and foods with a higher fat content or those containing harder-to-digest fats, and those rich in dietary sulfur, as garlic, egg yolks, and cruciferous vegetables.

You'll learn more about these four **Wildatarian** types in Chapter 3: What Type of **Wildatarian** Are You?

WILDATARIAN RECIPES

At the end of this book, you will find recipes I have created and tailored for each major type of **Wildatarian**. These recipes draw flavors from many cultures, including my own native Cuban heritage and my family's Spanish roots. As a Cuban refugee, I learned that food should never be wasted, and this is a tenet of the **Wildatarian** approach. I will also teach you how to use extra ingredients to make what I call convertible meals—using leftovers from one recipe to create another **Wildatarian** meal! You also can choose to be a sea-based **Wildatarian** and only consume fish and shellfish or become a plant-based **Wildatarian** with our yummy recipes for legumes, grains, nuts, seeds, fruits and vegetables.

RECIPES AND AFFIRMATIONS

The **Wildatarian** approach considers that *how you eat* matters as much as *what you eat*. The featured recipes are paired with affirmations and explanations of how the ingredients work synergistically to support immune function. Having this information available each time you prepare the recipe will help establish health-promoting thoughts and behaviors at the subconscious level.

STORIES OF TRANSFORMATION

The appendix highlights several Stories of Transformation from my practice to illustrate how the **Wildatarian** approach has changed lives. Take Glenn, whose amyloidosis and cancer were rebalanced. Or Erica, whose health issues associated with Lyme disease are no longer controlling her life. Madelyn, a teenage swim phenom, came to see us to reverse her alopecia totalis. We helped her to not only get her hair back but also to improve her swimming statistics with an eye toward the Olympic games.

For our clients who were "healthy" but wanted to optimize their health, the **Wildatarian** approach also created impactful improvements—for example, a retired international rugby player who wanted to get back into professional-level shape or an 18 year old pre-Olympic male swimmer who wanted to gain strength and cut time in the water. Both of these men achieved their goals in just a few months by following the **Wildatarian** lifestyle. These are not specifically highlighted in the Stories of Transformation but I share them to illustrate that anyone can benefit from adopting this approach.

Whether you are a:

- Crossfit junkie whose goal is to get shredded;
- Couple wondering why it is so difficult to conceive;
- Mom who is worried one of her three children will become diabetic;
- Teenage girl who is wondering why her periods are irregular and she keeps gaining weight;
- Middle-aged man who is tired, foggy-headed, suffers from digestive problems, and just can't seem to shed those last few pounds; or a
- Seemingly healthy person...

This book is for you!

No matter what your unique health concerns are, **Wildatarianism** is a path to a healthy, vibrant life full of energy, vitality, and mental clarity.

THE BOOK ROADMAP

This book provides an easy roadmap to a **Wildatarian** lifestyle.

CHAPTER 1: FROM MARKET TO TABLE addresses our evolutionary connections with food and the factors in today's commercial agriculture that challenge this connection. It speaks to the energetic currency in food and its relationship with our thoughts. You will also learn that how you eat is as important as what you eat.

CHAPTER 2: WILDATARIANISM: AN EASY PATH TO HEALTH will show you that this lifestyle is affordable and accessible. You will learn how to eat out and where to buy food. You will see that this lifestyle can fit into your life with minimal effort.

CHAPTER 3: WHAT TYPE OF WILDATARIAN ARE YOU? will help you figure out which of the four **Wildatarian** types represents you. Your type will guide the foods you eat for both the short term and the long term.

CHAPTER 4: FROM NATURE TO DENATURED will discuss some of the biggest dietary culprits involved in today's epidemic of disease and poor health. Understanding how and why the food you eat is detracting from health should help you sustain vibrancy in the future.

CHAPTERS 5–7 focus on different categories of food—proteins, grains, legumes, and others. This is where you will learn how and why the **Wildatarian** diet recommends certain types of food and asks you to abstain from others.

CHAPTER 8–10: RECIPES are mouthwatering, easy-to-prepare creations. Each recipe includes a key to adjusting ingredients so you can enjoy them based on your **Wildatarian** type.

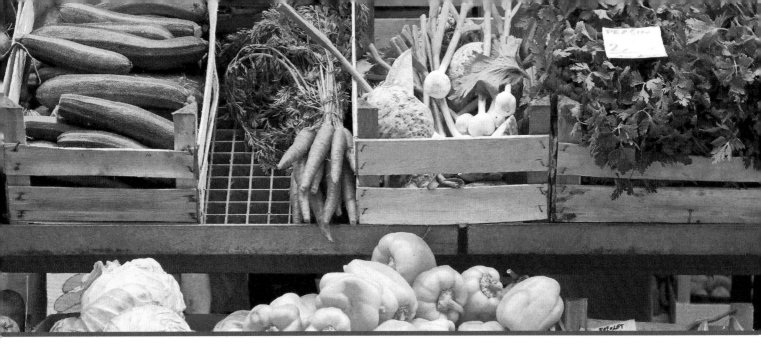

CHAPTER 1

THE MAKINGS OF A WILDATARIAN: FROM MARKET TO TABLE

Everything on this earth—including food—vibrates with kinetic energy. Energy is the building block of all matter. Because everything has energy, everything you think, eat, touch, and with which you come into contact can serve to either provide energetic support or deplete you of energy.

Your body makes chemical and electromagnetic exchanges when performing its daily functions. The foods you eat can generate healthy chemical responses, such as transforming healthy fats into energy for the brain, or unhealthy chemical responses, such as the body's attempt to break down and metabolize glyphosates (a synthetic crop herbicide), which may contribute to neurotoxicity and gut-brain imbalance. Electromagnetic responses can also result from the consumption of food. For example, coconut water, which is highly alkalizing and provides electrolytes necessary for neurotransmission and healthy mood, may help to promote a sense of calm and well-being. Conversely, refined sugar can create an energetic imbalance that spikes stress hormones because of its negative impact on insulin.

ENERGETIC CURRENCY OF DOMESTICATED ANIMAL PRODUCTION

Our demand for convenience has led to the commercialization of animal and dairy production, which has been tied to deleterious effects on our ever-declining health. These modern farming practices create sick and malnourished animals. It is well known that commercially produced animal products contain much fewer fat-soluble vitamins (such as A, D, E, and K) and less of the healthy fats (such as omega-3's) than their local, pasture-raised counterparts.

There have been many books written about the exposure of commercially-raised animals to high antibiotic and hormone loads. One of my personally most impactful reads was *The Omnivore's Dilemma*, written by Michael Pollan in 2006. Widely prevalent feeding methods run counter to evolutionary biology—they feature corn and soy, which animals cannot digest. Commercially raised animals lead stressful lives—crowded together in inhumane conditions, not allowed to move freely, and often maimed for convenience. All of this results in significant negative and unhealthy consequences at the biological and genetic levels—both for these animals and for us. When we consume products from these animals, we essentially consume their stress. Chickens and cows in an inflamed/stressed state are at increased risk for amyloid (less digestible, misfolded protein) formation.

Alternatively, when we eat foods local to our area, and those humanely raised to be lower in amyloids, we reduce the risk of exposing our system to harmful chemical and energetic byproducts. Additionally, because sustainable farming methods avoid harmful chemicals, antibiotics, and unsuitable feed, the resulting food carries a greater nutrient value—providing ample energetic currency for our bodies to use.

HOW YOU EAT MATTERS AS MUCH AS WHAT YOU EAT

Your energetic connection with food begins the moment you make food choices, whether you are at the grocery store, a farmers market, a restaurant, or even in your kitchen.

Eating in a relaxed emotional state increases stomach acid production, which contributes to your health in the following ways:

- Aids protein digestion
- Liberates digestive enzymes for the breakdown of fats, proteins, and sugars
- Enhances peristalsis (a series of wave-like muscle contractions that move food along the digestive tract and assist in the complex process of digestion)

Conversely, when you eat in a state of stress, your digestion is impaired. You produce less stomach acid and fewer enzymes, and peristalsis is slowed.

In response to high stress, the body will crave some sugar or fat to replenish the energy it is lacking. This leads us to gravitate toward "comfort" foods, which are typically high in inflammatory ingredients such as unhealthy fats, refined sugars, preservatives, hormones, amyloids, and synthetic chemicals. *This is a recipe for disaster.*

Dr. Candace Pert, past professor in the Department of Physiology and Biophysics at Georgetown University's School of Medicine and author of *Molecules of Emotion: The Science Behind Mind-Body Medicine*, helps us understand the power that our mind has over the physical body. She describes how thoughts and feelings directly and profoundly affect our health and well-being. This new science illuminates that we are one system integrated at a molecular level, so treating the physical body separately from the emotional state is not sensible.

EATING MINDFULLY

This mind-body connection is why I encourage you to start an *intentional* relationship with your food. Often, we find ourselves eating *mindlessly*—eating while watching television, reading the newspaper, involved in an argument, or in the car on the way to work. Remind yourself that when you eat mindlessly, you reduce your capacity to break down, assimilate, and digest your meal. Although it may not be possible to completely avoid these habits, you can increase your level of awareness to foster eating mindfully.

HEALING RECIPES

Following your **Wildatarian** diet, you'll find a variety of delicious recipes for foods with carefully chosen ingredients that work independently and synergistically to promote healing.

I created my recipes very intentionally. As I was preparing these recipes for the book, I honored the space in which I was creating them. I brought elements of nature into the space with flowers, candles, natural light, and herbs. I infused them with love. Each recipe was inspired, prepared, and photographed in the same manner in which I wish for you to have a relationship with food.

For example, in my *Mediterranean-Style Quinoa Salad*, I share inspirational insights about the beauty of the dish, its quick prep time (it takes less than fifteen minutes to prepare), and how its nutritional benefits will make *you* feel on the inside. This is powerful language. I emphasize that this vegetarian meal is a complete protein loaded with manganese, magnesium, iron, copper, and phosphorus, which helps to combat the health problems that our Standard American Lifestyle actively works to create. I describe how chickpeas prevent blood sugar levels from rising too rapidly and how their high molybdenum content may help in detoxifying sulfites. Sulfites, which are often used as food preservatives, can contribute to oxidative stress and have been linked to ADHD, asthma, and allergies.

CONNECTION BETWEEN YOUR FOOD AND YOUR WORDS

Why is this important? Because as you make the meal and you read through the recipe, it will remind you and your cells of the nutritional benefits of the dish. It is a form of neuro-linguistic programming, which is an approach to communication where, based on the language we use, connections between neurological processes can shift behavioral patterns and beliefs. As you learn that these recipes have powerful properties, your brain affirms it and your cells receive the information.

Each recipe also is paired with an affirmation. Supportive affirmations provide an element of repetition that allows positive thoughts to establish themselves at a deeper level. Ultimately, positive affirmations have the power to shift negative beliefs and behaviors that are barriers to healthy living.

Just before you begin your meal, take several deep breaths; this will increase your oxygenation and stimulate cellular function. Experience your food with a level of awareness, knowing that you are participating in the process of the transformation of matter into energy for use by your cells. Chew your food slowly and thoroughly, experiencing the taste, smell, and texture of each bite. This will aid in digestion and assimilation.

MEALS AND MENU PLANNING

Meals and menu planning are integral to converting to a **Wildatarian** lifestyle. If you don't have an executable, tactical plan, all the knowledge and information will not yield results. Take photos of your grocery lists and recipes and keep them on your phone so you have them with you at all times. One hour of planning can save you countless hours of food preparation and shopping. You can turn your fridge and pantry into healthy "fast-food" establishments if you plan ahead!

Much of eating healthfully is to have a weekly plan and execute it. It never works to be standing in front of the refrigerator before dinner trying to figure out what you will make that night. I counsel my clients to look at their calendar and adjust meals to the activities for the week. (That's what I do!) I'm also a fan of using a slow cooker: it takes less than five minutes to assemble all the ingredients and then let this kitchen helper do the rest.

If your schedule is filled with busy, activity-filled evenings, then either prep your meal in the morning before work or plan ahead and make soups, chilis, and grilled wild meats such as bison, duck, lamb, or Cornish game hen—these can be prepared easily in minutes and paired with a salad for those busy nights. While I am getting ready for work in the morning, I roast zucchini and yellow squash, which take just a few minutes. In the evening, after dinner I often roast sweet potatoes, winter squash, or other veggies that take a bit more roasting time. These yummy, prepared veggies can be used for future meals when time is scarce.

CONVERTIBLE RECIPES

The convertible recipes in this book make it fast and easy to repurpose previously made meals into something new. *Herb-Rubbed Roasted Duck* can be converted into quesadillas, barbecue sandwiches, or a duck, cucumber, and goat feta salad—and then soup from the carcass. Just combine a bag of frozen organic veggies and a can of beans with the stock made from the already seasoned carcass, and voila!

The **Wildatarian** recipes included make menu planning and meals doable. Having an executable plan lowers the stress response. It can be done with ease. So simple, so delicious, so nourishing, so organized!

With the awareness of food and self, you may gain a level of control and achieve freedom from the uncertainties of stress, illness, and ailment. Ultimately, it is this freedom that is at the root of the **Wildatarian** lifestyle, establishing the ***Tru of You***.

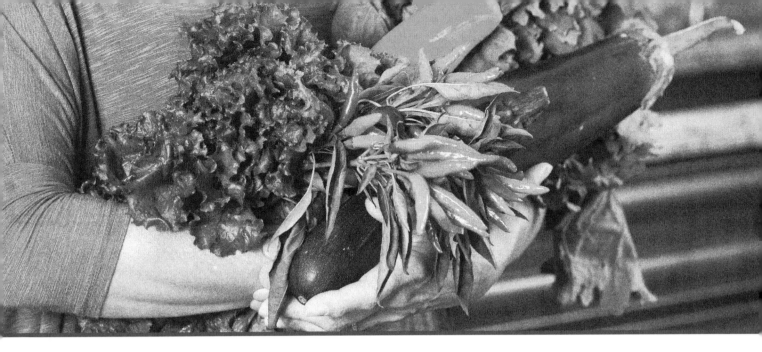

CHAPTER 2

WILDATARIANISM: AN EASY PATH TO HEALTH

Becoming a **Wildatarian** and living a **Wildatarian** lifestyle are not about deprivation. Instead, this lifestyle focuses on abundance and bounty in foods and attitudes that serve *you*. The long-standing approach of focusing on calorie-counting, carbohydrate-to-fat ratios, or one-size-fits-all dietary prescriptions has failed to improve our state of health. I believe that if you feed the body what it needs—by understanding your genetic predispositions coupled with your current state of health—you can increase healthy energy levels, obtain relief from autoimmune conditions or gut imbalances, increase your ability to learn and thrive in your school or work environment, enjoy healthy fertility, and revel in a general sense of well-being. What you eat, breathe, drink, feel, and think has the power to alter your physical body and all aspects of your health. These things also have the power to change the expression of your genes, meaning how your genes work to keep you from or move you to health.

When you think about the word *diet*, I encourage you to think about approaching it in a completely different way. I have redefined "diet" to move it from a low-vibration, fear-based, deprivation-state word to one oriented around abundance and mindfulness. Diet should include everything that we consume in life, not just our food. Diet is how we consume and assimilate our thoughts and how we consume the environment around us, *as well as how we consume and assimilate our food*. This consumption should be oriented toward gratitude, nourishment, and assimilation, and that is what the **Wildatarian** diet and lifestyle represent.

On your **Wildatarian** journey, you will focus on the Big Three of protein, fat, and sulfur malabsorption. You will nourish your body with a more easily assimilated source of animal protein—wild game, which is generally leaner, higher in beneficial, anti-inflammatory fats, lower in cholesterol, and richer in minerals than their domesticated counterparts. You will choose grains, nuts, and seeds rich in minerals and fiber, which help support a healthy gut biome and balance blood glucose. You will consume legumes that are easily digestible proteins and choose those that are low in mycotoxin[2] content and rich in antioxidants. You will indulge in healthy sugars—those that do not tax your endocrine organs or disrupt your stress response. **Wildatarian** is a powerful approach to health and healing.

You can be a **Wildatarian** at any age, at any stage, and anywhere. Moms have started making homemade **Wildatarian** baby meals. Our teenage clients have embraced this approach and manage it handily even in their high school and college environments. The following is a Facebook post from one of my college-age clients:

> *My saving grace Teri Cochrane—figured out what was wrong with me and helped me learn to avoid the foods that I couldn't break down and that were causing my body to fight against me, which allowed me to reach the healthiest point ever in my entire life. After which, a medical setback re-triggered my inability to break down domesticated animal proteins and fats, and pushed me back to square one ... so back I went to the Wildatarian approach. Today, I am a gluten-free, Wildatarian girl who loves and enjoys every day of having a healthy relationship with food and exercise.*

Even our older clients embrace this lifestyle as they regain their vitality.

---

2 Mycotoxins are fungal metabolites which may feed unwanted pathogens such as candida, strep, staph, and other small intestinal bacteria, which can disrupt the integrity and balance of our gut biome and which may promote amyloid formation.

PLANT-BASED WILDATARIAN

There are many ways to be a **Wildatarian**. If you don't eat meat or fish, you can still participate in the **Wildatarian** diet and lifestyle by being a plant-based **Wildatarian**.

I respect all kinds of eating styles, including vegetarian and vegan. Just because the **Wildatarian** philosophy advocates for the consumption of game and other more "wild" animals, you don't have to eat them. If you follow a vegan or vegetarian eating philosophy, you have already removed a big concern the **Wildatarian** diet is trying to address: not eating animals means you are avoiding a possible source of amyloids and other broken or misfolded proteins.

But you are not totally out of the woods. If vegetarian or vegan, you are likely consuming gluten, a protein that has been made virtually indigestible by our farming practices. You are also probably eating many foods rich in mycotoxins and molds (more on that in Chapter 6: **Wildatarian** Grains). You may also be eating foods like peanuts, which are a known source of aflatoxin, a dangerous mold byproduct linked to cancer and other diseases. If you are vegetarian, you could be eating cow dairy, which may be a problematic food for you.

The bottom line is that the **Wildatarian** philosophy is flexible enough to accommodate you regardless of whether you choose to eat animals or not. If you are vegan, please learn about some likely nutrient deficiencies associated with your eating style, and supplement where necessary.

HEALTHY *AND* AFFORDABLE

The **Wildatarian** lifestyle can be affordable. Wild game may be a few dollars more per pound than commercially raised meat and fish, but the health benefits it imparts may result in possible savings from less prescription medication and lowered healthcare costs down the road. I call it a *short-term investment in your long-term health goals*. You can significantly lower your per-pound cost by incorporating beans with the animal meat. Two cans of beans per one pound of wild game will lower your price per pound by more than half.

Another way to save on food dollars is by eating at home more often. This is in line with the **Wildatarian** lifestyle of using leftovers so nothing is wasted or thrown away. Eating at home saves on gas and, therefore, reduces the carbon footprint of your meal.

If you do decide to eat out, focus on being a solution seeker. It is now easy to preview menus of the restaurants you plan on patronizing. Restaurant dining has become **Wildatarian** friendly. Bison and buffalo are becoming very popular and can be found when dining out. You also can find lamb, fish, and shellfish on most restaurant menus. Beans and rice are also good menu options if you are a plant-based **Wildatarian**. You also can ask for customized meals that meet your dietary needs. I travel often and manage to find **Wildatarian** fare everywhere I go, without exception. Even national food chains such as Panera, Chipotle, and Silver Diner are moving toward healthful eating where you can find a variety of **Wildatarian** options.

If you find yourself in a scenario where **Wildatarian** meat is not an option, I recommend you avoid the least-desirable options. Chicken may be the most unhealthy non-Wild protein you can consume, so beef may be the better choice. Or choose to have wild-caught fish and seafood (farm-raised fish come with extras you don't want to be putting in your body; more on farmed fish later in this book), or choose beans and rice and avoid the dilemma altogether.

You can find wild meat, fish, and foul selections at most larger grocers. The typical **Wildatarian** meats you will find at mainstream stores include bison, buffalo, lamb, Cornish game hen, duck, wild fish, and shellfish. Chains such as Costco, Food Lion, Giant, Harris Teeter, Kroger, and Publix as well as Trader Joe's and Whole Foods offer them. You also can find these at many of your local farmers markets. Look for wild boar, pheasant, venison, elk, and other wild cuts at smaller specialty stores. Having a friend or family member who hunts is another fabulous option. One of my staff members is a hunter and often shares cuts of wild boar that she hunts.

Preparing wild cuts of meat may appear to be difficult because they are so lean. Yes, this meat is generally lower in fat, but my cooking methods conserve the delicious juices. I find that these meats can be very buttery if prepared properly. A slow cooker or a pressure cooker are great kitchen appliances that ensure a juicy, tender, and tasty result. Additionally, my recipes are created with rich flavors that eliminate the potential gamey flavor. Many of my clients say that once they try bison or buffalo, they prefer it to beef. The same holds true for pheasant and wild boar.

In Chapter 5: Protective Proteins, you will notice that I include some non-WILD meats in the **Wildatarian** program. I am referring specifically to lamb, duck and Cornish game hen. Our program allows these specific animal products for several reasons. We look at animal meats on a spectrum. Wild game is best, followed by heritage cuts and then grass-fed. My goal for you is to stay on the wilder end of the spectrum, but I know that it may not always be possible. My clinical outcomes show that you'll receive maximum health benefits as long as the majority of the meats you consume are wild.

Research has shown amyloids from commercially raised cattle can induce an amyloid disease state in inflamed mice.

Our clinical practice has shown that most individuals can consume lamb, duck, and Cornish game hen without experiencing amyloid-induced symptoms.

Because lamb, duck and Cornish game hen comprise a comparatively small percentage of meats raised and consumed, their genetic and inflammatory status may be superior to that of their amyloid-rich cousins. Please keep in mind that this may not be the case at some point in the future, when the conditions under which these animals are raised deteriorate to a point that makes them amyloid-rich and highly inflammatory.

While truly wild meats are lower in fat than their counterparts, lamb, duck, and Cornish game hen are not, if you choose varieties raised under healthy conditions, they will likely contain inflammation-lowering fats that are considered beneficial.

The **Wildatarian** approach is a lifestyle. It is a pledge you make with yourself to live your life more naturally, to purchase and consume foods that are whole and pure. You are a reflection of what you put into your body. When you choose whole foods in the purest state, you affirm the greater connections with your community and your planet. It is a commitment to personal engagement.

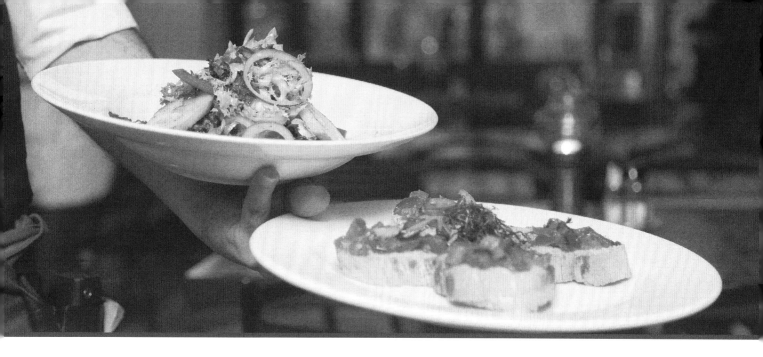

CHAPTER 3

WHAT TYPE OF WILDATARIAN ARE YOU?

Bio-individuality is a cornerstone of my practice. The term *bio-individuality*, which includes our distinct genetic fingerprint, underscores that the nutritional and chemical makeup of each person is unique. Biochemical individuality (also known as bio-individuality) is a term coined by Dr. Roger Williams, who discovered vitamin B5 (pantothenic acid). He also first isolated and named folic acid, another B vitamin.

Dietary and other needs vary from person to person. People have unique profiles due to their genetic makeup and environment, but these profiles can change over time. In essence, what may be good for me may be awful for you, and vice versa. What may be nourishing in your healthy state may be depleting when you are sick or vulnerable. Therefore, certain foods may not be optimal for your genetics and your current state of health.

Reflecting on the countless clients I have seen through my years in practice, and taking into account my ongoing research, I have created four types of **Wildatarian**s based on the **Wildatarian** Big Three: *protein, fat, and sulfur malabsorption.* Each of the four is based on the idea that dietary amyloids should be avoided as much as possible.

The four types are:

- **W–TYPE Wildatarian™** Basic
- **WF–TYPE Wildatarian™** (Low-Fat)
- **WS–TYPE Wildatarian™** (Low-Sulfur)
- **WFS–TYPE Wildatarian™** (Low-Fat and Low-Sulfur)

I developed these **Wildatarian** types to help you consume foods that are optimal for your body. At the root of it all is your gut—a pathway connecting the mouth to the rectum. When functioning at optimal capacity, our gut works as a bouncer, only letting in what is helpful and nourishing. The gut has to have integrity—the barrier has to be smart enough and tight enough to perform its functions. If your gut is leaky or permeable[3], pathogens such as yeast, bacteria, viruses, parasites, and amyloids can interfere with optimal digestion and actually break through the intestinal barrier that protects the rest of your body.

I have coined the term **HealAndSeal™** to describe a state where we create a gut biome and gut barrier function that has integrity, where we balance our intestinal population of bacteria and viruses, reducing the likelihood of unfavorable molecules passing through the intestinal barrier to other parts of the body. **HealAndSeal** promotes better immune function and health.

It is important that you consume an adequate amount of the types of proteins that your body can break down and assimilate based on your genome and health state—and remember that each person's needs are slightly different. The truth is that some "healthy" proteins are most likely contributing to the dysfunction you may be feeling, because your individual biochemistry is not designed to healthfully consume them.

HOW TO DETERMINE YOUR BIO-INDIVIDUAL NEEDS

I have provided an online quiz to help you determine your bio-individual **Wildatarian** type. After you take the quiz and establish your **Wildatarian** type, you will understand the foods your

---

3   Leaky or permeable means the intestinal barrier is no longer selectively permeable or that it may allow pathogens or larger molecules to pass through. Our immune system, not recognizing these molecules, may consider them an invader to the body and respond through inflammation or even antibodies. This sets the stage for autoimmunity.

body is best equipped to assimilate, break down, and absorb. The questions are easy to answer and pertain to common and observable traits associated with your body, such as the frequency and consistency of your bowel habits, your body composition, or medical conditions you have been diagnosed with. Find the quiz at tericochrane.com/quiz. My **Wildatarian** approach removes many commercially raised animal products from your food plate, no matter what type of **Wildatarian** you are. Even if your quiz results reveal that you don't need to limit protein, sulfur, or fat, I still recommend you follow the **W–TYPE Wildatarian** Basic plan.

IMPLEMENTATION OF THE WILDATARIAN EATING PLAN

When implementing the **Wildatarian** eating plan, I recommend two phases: the **Rebalance** phase and the **Maintenance** phase. This book provides information to start your **Wildatarian** journey, and you can learn more about both phases through the **HealAndSeal** program at tericochrane.com. The **Rebalance** phase lasts about six weeks. During this phase, you will avoid foods that may not best serve your type, and instead you will focus on foods that your body may be more easily able to assimilate. The **Maintenance** phase is the way of eating you will sustain for the long term—it is specific to your physiology. In this phase, you will slowly reintroduce some of the eliminated foods to determine if your body can tolerate them. Using trial and error, and listening to your body, you will be able to determine the most ideal way of eating for your unique bio-individuality.

I include a full sampling of **Wildatarian** recipes that tell how you will substitute ingredients to meet the needs of your **Wildatarian** type. Chapters 5–10 provide guidelines for foods to avoid and which foods to steer toward. The **HealAndSeal** program contains a detailed listing of the foods that may be consumed liberally, those that should be moderately consumed, and those that must be avoided during each of these phases.

W–TYPE Wildatarian Basic: The **W–TYPE** eliminates gluten and beef, pork/ham, chicken, and turkey. As previously mentioned, we now know that commercially raised animal products may not be the healthiest food source. The amyloids and dysfunctional proteins contained in these foods may contribute to protein malabsorption. Everyone should strive to follow a **Wildatarian**

approach, even those who are able to process protein, because of the multiple health benefits this approach offers. All **Wildatarian** types will avoid these potentially destructive foods.

Some signs of protein malabsorption include the following symptomatology:

- Trouble building muscles
- Ligament laxity
- Lightheadedness
- Burping after eating
- Grey pallor
- Undigested food in stool
- Gluten sensitivity
- Fullness hours after eating
- Constipation
- Ammonia-smelling urine or sweat
- Dark urine
- Elevated protein in urine as determined by a urine test
- Kidney disease

Consult individual recipes to see if they can be used during your **Rebalance** phase. If you are a **W–TYPE**, then you will be able to consume every recipe in this book during your **Maintenance** phase.

WF–TYPE Wildatarian (Low-Fat): When following the **Wildatarian** diet, you will eliminate gluten, beef, pork/ham, chicken, and turkey. In addition, if you are the **WF–TYPE**, you will avoid foods with a higher fat content or those containing harder-to-digest fats.

Dietary fat provides the fuel our bodies need for functions such as brain health, hormone production, and cell membrane integrity. Cell membranes are made up of fats we have consumed over the previous months, and our ability to use the fat we ingest will either create a cell membrane that is bouncy and functional or leave it brittle and inefficient.

Fortunately, the indiscriminate vilification of all dietary fat has been debunked by recent medical research. But when your body cannot break this fat down and assimilate it, the benefits of healthy constituents such as omega-3s and monounsaturated fatty acids are not fully available to you. In fact, if you become fat malabsorbed—unable to process fats—you may increase the burden on many of your body's systems and promote dysfunction such as gut permeability, clogged liver, impaired hormone metabolism, and acne. Some telltale signs of fat malabsorption include:

- Changes in stool to light color, floating, "fuzzy," and greasy
- Strong body odor
- Bumps on the back of the arms
- Acne
- Yellowish skin tone
- Very dry skin
- Hormonal imbalances such as polycystic ovary syndrome (PCOS), premenstrual syndrome (PMS), or premenstrual dysphoric disorder
- Edema
- Diarrhea
- Nausea or excessive fullness after eating
- Gallbladder pain (right side under ribs)
- Right scapula pain (referred gallbladder pain)
- Gallstones
- Gallbladder removal

The **WF–TYPE** avoids high-fat nuts, high-fat fish, and even higher-fat **Wildatarian** meats. Be cognizant of fatty ingredients in some recipes, and make substitutions as necessary.

WS–TYPE Wildatarian (Low-Sulfur): When following the **Wildatarian** diet, you will eliminate gluten, beef, pork/ham, chicken, and turkey. In addition, if you are the **WS–TYPE**, avoid foods rich in dietary sulfur, such as egg yolks, some shellfish, garlic, and cruciferous vegetables. This holds true, even though these foods are widely touted as tremendously healthy.

Foods rich in sulfur—an important compound—are some of the healthiest foods around. They include well-known health promoters such as garlic, cruciferous vegetables (including kale, broccoli, and cauliflower), and egg yolks. Dietary sulfur is important to many of our body's systems, including detoxification, digestive integrity, cancer-fighting ability, and oxidation reduction. Brassicas—members of the cruciferous vegetable family—contain a host of phytonutrients, including indole-3-carbinol, which helps keep our livers clear and opposes hormone-induced cancers. Cabbage is full of the amino acid L-glutamine—a key nutrient in digestive maintenance and repair.

Unfortunately, as a result of the potential key benefits of these foods, many of us may be over-sulfured, because we consume too much dietary sulfur for our genetics. Several popular dietary plans encourage us to consume as many sulfur-containing foods as possible. Juicing with sulfur-rich compounds, such as kale and cabbage, is very common. While this dietary advice may be fine for many of us, those with expressed genetic vulnerabilities in sulfur metabolism will not benefit from these dietary practices. A short-term abstention from sulfur-rich compounds is a key element of the **WS–TYPE** plan.

Eliminating cruciferous vegetables may be difficult, especially for those of us who consider a diet bountiful in vegetables to be a healthy one. Onions are considered sulfuric, but even if you are a **WS–TYPE,** we allow them when cooked. This is because cooking onions greatly lowers their sulfur content. I do, however, ask you to stay away from raw onions.

Some telltale signs of sulfur sensitivity include:

- Allergies to sulfa-containing medications
- Reactions to either red or white wine
- Reactions to garlic
- Reactions to eggs
- Asthma or wheezing after ingesting food, especially dried fruit or foods with preservatives
- Strong urine odor after eating asparagus
- Arthritis
- Joint pain

- Bursitis or tendonitis
- Parkinson's disease
- Crohn's disease
- Ulcerative colitis
- Irritable bowel
- Attention deficit hyperactivity disorder (ADHD)
- Calcifications, including neuromas or lipomas
- Certain neurotransmitter imbalances, such as dopamine, epinephrine, and serotonin
- Some skin rashes, including psoriasis

If you need to limit sulfur, you may need to omit or substitute ingredients in some **Wildatarian** recipes. For example, omit garlic or substitute bell pepper for the garlic in *Cuban Black Beans*, and this dish will be perfectly acceptable for the **WS–TYPE**.

Some recipes crafted for the **WS–TYPE** include small amounts of sulfuric compounds. Because the concentration is quite low and there are other ingredients that mitigate the effects of the sulfuric compounds on your body, we consider these compounds to be safe for this type's consumption.

Omitting sulfur-rich foods from your diet does not have to be forever, but it does provide your body a break from a food source that it cannot easily metabolize. As you continue to **HealAndSeal**, you will be able to enjoy most of the sulfuric ingredients in the recipes. One way to know you are sensitive to sulfur is to reintroduce it. If your symptoms reappear, continue to avoid these foods.

WFS–TYPE Wildatarian (Low-Fat and Low-Sulfur): When following the **Wildatarian** diet, you will eliminate gluten, beef, pork/ham, chicken, and turkey. If you are the **WFS–TYPE**, you also will avoid both higher fat and higher sulfur-containing ingredients in foods and recipes. This type is most restrictive, because it combines the limitations in the **WF** and **WS** approach. Examples of the foods you will eliminate include high-fat nuts, high-fat animal protein, garlic, and cruciferous vegetables. Please refer to the **WF-TYPE** and **WS-TYPE** sections above for more information, but you will still have a bounty of options with healthy and easily digestible fats, including seeds such as sunflower, pumpkin and flax, as well as healthy vegetables such as spinach greens, squashes, sweet potatoes, and avocados.

GUIDELINES FOR ALL WILDATARIAN TYPES IN CHOOSING PLAN-APPROVED RECIPES

This book provides many tasty, healthy, and easy-to-make recipes. However, not all recipes are appropriate for each of the **Wildatarian** types and phases. To help you decide if a recipe can be used for your particular plan, consult the **applicability to food plans** table included with each recipe. A sample is included below. In this particular table, the **W–TYPE** can use the recipe as written, the **WS** and **WFS** types should remove the garlic, and the **WF** and **WFS** types should use buffalo as the meat of choice and coconut milk beverage as a lower-fat option.

APPLICABILITY TO FOOD PLANS

W	• Use recipe as is
WS	• Eliminate garlic from recipe
WF	• Use buffalo (bison) as your meat of choice • Substitute coconut milk beverage for full-fat coconut milk
WFS	• Eliminate garlic from recipe • Use buffalo (bison) as your meat of choice • Substitute coconut milk beverage for full-fat coconut milk

The next section of this book dives into each of the major food groups as I define them. It explains the benefits as well as the injurious properties of different types of food and educates you in distinguishing which ones are best suited for you. We delve into the science of how and why our food supply is changing and what we can do to counter this unfortunate trend.

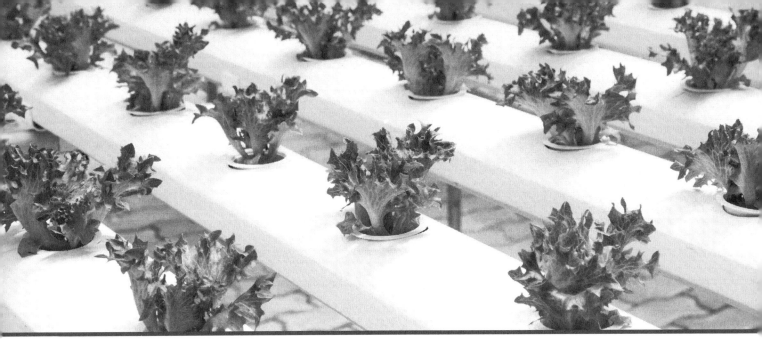

CHAPTER 4

FROM BALANCE TO IMBALANCE: LOSING OUR CONNECTION TO NATURE

How did we get here? How did we become an obese nation, with a growing epidemic of autoimmune disease and cancer, and one crippled by health care costs? How can it be that for the first time in history, children are projected to have a shorter lifespan than their parents?

Food used to come from the Source, from the earth, complete with all the nutrients needed for life. Our planet, including its air, water, soil, and natural lunar and solar cycles, was created with everything we needed to survive and thrive—in an unadulterated form. As members of early civilization, humans recognized their link to the forces and cycles of the earth. They shared a natural connection to and reverence for food, because for the most part, they grew or gathered their own and ate for sustenance and health. They knew how and when to plant seeds for harvest, how to rotate crops so different vitamins and minerals would be drawn into the seedlings from the nutrient-rich soil, and when to pick the food for maximum nutritional value. This may have been the original and truly sustainable form of farming. A spiritual connection between food and the way it was grown, prepared, and consumed was a natural part of the rhythm of life.

FAILINGS OF THE STANDARD AMERICAN DIET (SAD)

Today, things are quite different. Many people believe that the food they eat gives the body what it needs to function, but in the Western world, most of us are overfed and obese yet undernourished. Our standard food supply is not only devoid of nutrients but also harmful to us and our earth—this is SAD, the Standard American Diet. This diet has been linked to an exponential increase in many chronic illnesses and the obesity epidemic in children and adults.

We live with blind trust that our regulatory agencies and agricultural systems are producing safe, sustainable, and nutritious food. However, today's food is grown with the use of synthetic chemicals and from genetically modified seeds. Western agriculture has tinkered with nature's bounty in its pursuit of greater efficiency, higher yields, and convenience.

Our standard, off-the-shelf supermarket food does not offer enough in basic nutrition. While we certainly get an immediate boost from that sugary "health" drink or bar, bag of snacks, or boxed dinner, few of us wonder why we crash with low energy levels and mental fogginess just twenty minutes later. Not enough of us understand that in many cases, the SAD is actually depleting the body of what it needs. SAD is lacking in vital vitamins, minerals, and nutrients that are essential for growth, repair, and maintenance of cellular function. The **Wildatarian** lifestyle will show you that convenience does not have to come at the sacrifice of nutrition.

EFFECTS OF CHEMICALS AND GENETIC MODIFICATION

The practice of growing only one type of agricultural product on the same large plot of land year after year—*monocropping*—is standard practice. This technique reduces the need for human labor required to grow food, but it comes at a great cost of nutrient-depleted soil, and, as a result, nutrient-depleted food. Monocropping also increases the vulnerability of plants to insects, fungi, and pests, which then requires additional use of insecticides, fungicides, and herbicides. These poisons and hormone disruptors leach into our crops and pollute our water supply, creating potential environmental and public health hazards.

Vulnerable crops are genetically engineered to withstand ever-increasing amounts of sprayed chemicals needed to protect them against pests and insects, which creates a vicious cycle. Genetically modified organisms (GMOs) are taking over our food supply. The United States Department of Agriculture (USDA) reports that as of 2011, 94 percent of soybeans and 88 percent of corn grown in the United States are genetically modified.

CHEAPER ISN'T BETTER

Not only is genetically modified pseudo food easily available, but it is also relatively inexpensive. Interestingly, what we spend on food in proportion to our income has declined dramatically since 1960, according to data published by the U.S. Department of Agriculture. The average share of per capita income spent on food fell from 17.5 percent in 1960 to 9.9 percent in 2013. Our food is cheap, but it comes at a great cost to our health and environment, as we are now facing the largest epidemic of metabolic disorders ever in the history of our habitation on this planet.

We also are spending much less time in food preparation, because we eat out or purchase packaged foods to prepare at home. Foods should not come from a box with ingredients that cannot be pronounced.

The **Wildatarian** lifestyle combines convenience—a necessity in today's life—with wholesome nutrition through simple menu and meal planning. "Grab-and-go" and "wrap-and-roll" do not have to come from a restaurant or a store—they can be made in your own kitchen. Even the least experienced chef can practice food assembly, putting together a whole, nutritious meal from easy-to-use and healthy ingredients. If we build healthy habits of menu and meal planning, then "fast food" can come right from our kitchen, ready and available when time is short.

REFINED SUGAR: A MAJOR VILLAIN

Refined sugar, and more specifically high fructose corn syrup (HFCS), contributes to insulin resistance—a precursor to diabetes. Insulin resistance occurs when our cell membranes become resistant to the action of insulin, a hormone that escorts sugar into the cells to lower blood glucose levels. This results in high blood sugar and high blood insulin levels, which is a serious combination.

When you consume refined sugar and other highly processed convenience foods, your blood sugar spikes. Continued consumption strains the pancreas, because as blood sugar rises, the pancreas releases insulin to bring that sugar into the cells for use, thereby reducing circulating blood glucose. Repeated cycles of this can lead to blood glucose falling to below normal levels—causing a temporary hypoglycemic condition (low blood sugar). Hypoglycemia, in turn, stimulates hunger in an effort to bring blood sugar back to acceptable levels and causes cravings for sugary foods; eating more sugar once again spikes blood sugar levels. This restarts the blood sugar roller coaster anew.

Over time, cells become resistant to this important action of insulin. This means the cells no longer recognize the need to use circulating insulin to bring glucose into the cell, resulting in high insulin and high blood glucose levels. This cycle can have devastating effects as insulin resistance turns into hyperglycemia (high blood sugar) and Type 2 diabetes. With Type 1 diabetes, the body no longer creates beta cells (whose primary function is to store and release insulin), and external insulin is needed to manage blood sugar. With Type 2 diabetes, the body's beta cells still secrete insulin, but its cells become insulin resistant and need outside help to bring glucose into the cells to balance blood sugar.

Approximately 25 percent of our average caloric intake now comes from sugars, with fructose making up the largest share. The average U.S. consumer ingests more than 150 pounds of sugar annually, up from eleven pounds a century ago. Today, a seven-year-old could easily be consuming three times his or her body weight in sugar each year. This is partially fueled by soft drink consumption, where HFCS is the primary sweetener. Its consumption has doubled in the United States in the past ten years.

HIGH FRUCTOSE CORN SYRUP (HFCS)

Almost all nutritionists point to high fructose corn syrup (HFCS) consumption as a major culprit in the nation's obesity crisis and contributor to diabetes and insulin resistance. Most of the HFCS in the United States is made from genetically modified corn filled with pesticides, herbicides, mold, and mycotoxins.

HFCS is extremely soluble and mixes well, so you'll find it in many foods on your grocer's shelves. It is sweet, cheap to produce, and easy to store. It's used in everything from cereals to pasta sauces, ketchup, bacon, and beer. It is even used in so-called "health products" like protein bars and yogurts. HFCS is also the primary sweetener used in soft drinks, which are now readily available to children in school vending machines. Soft drink consumption trends are improving, but many other types of beverages that are replacing soda contain HFCS also. The best way to know what is in packaged goods is to read food labels. If HFCS is included in the ingredients, avoid that product.

According to statistics from the Centers for Disease Control and Prevention, one out of every three children born after the year 2000 is at risk of developing diabetes in their lifetime. Before 1980, children were seldom diagnosed with Type 2 diabetes. As of 2014, more than 200,000 children have been diagnosed. Manufacturers are ever more creative with their use and labeling of HFCS, hiding its presence behind benign-sounding acronyms. HFCS now can be legally labeled as fructose or fructose syrup, which sounds healthier. Today, more than ever, we must be our own detectives to ensure we are not inadvertently consuming this food source with toxic elements.

> I encourage you to follow my philosophy regarding food labeling: If you cannot read or pronounce the ingredient, then you should not be putting it into your body— *can't read it, won't eat it.*

PESTICIDES, HERBICIDES, AND XENOESTROGENS

Studies show that pesticides and herbicides may increase the risk of many cancers, chronic disease, and birth defects. Roughly 1.2 billion pounds of pesticides and herbicides are sprayed on or added to food crops in the United States annually. It is estimated that only 2 percent of the more than 600 pesticides currently used in the United States reduce pests on crops. The remaining 98 percent are leached into our water and absorbed into the air, and become part of our food supply.

The average American consumes five pounds of these toxins per year. Many are known carcinogens and can disrupt neurological and endocrine system function. Specifically, xenoestrogens are substances that mimic hormones in your body, leading to hormone imbalance. These toxins are stored in fatty tissue, making their detoxification more difficult. The more fatty tissue you have, the more toxins you store. Traditional and domesticated animal meat and dairy products have extremely high concentrations of these toxins as well, because the animals eat chemically treated feed, which accumulates in their tissues. More about this in Chapter 5.

To help you make better selections when buying produce, the Environmental Working Group compiles an annual list of the top offenders of pesticide-contaminated fruits and vegetables called the Dirty Dozen. Typical offenders include berries, peaches, soft squash, celery, and apples. Know what you are eating. Choose organic when possible, or at least steer clear of the foods carrying the heaviest toxic load.

PRESERVATIVES AND FOOD DYES

Preservatives, synthetic food dyes, and artificial flavorings should be avoided, especially if you have food sensitivities, allergies, asthma, migraines, ADHD, depression, or anxiety. These substances are added to food to enhance appearance and increase shelf life. They offer no nutritional value and have been linked to many deleterious health conditions.

SULFITES AND OTHER PRESERVATIVES keep dried fruit fresh and soft and are often added to wine and beer for freshness. They can provoke attacks in those with asthma and may increase the chances of developing autoimmune digestive disorders like Crohn's disease, ulcerative colitis, and leaky gut in certain individuals. Most lunch meats, ham, and bacon are preserved with sodium nitrates, which convert to nitrous acid in the stomach and may increase the risk of stomach cancer. These preservatives have been banned in Germany and Norway, but the USDA continues to allow their use. In addition, formaldehyde may be added to frozen vegetables as a disinfectant.

ALUMINUM, also used as a preservative, has been linked to dementia and thyroid dysfunction. It can leach into our food when used in food packaging (like colas), and is also added to baking powder, antacids, and many antiperspirants.

ARTIFICIAL COLORS AND DYES fill the foods that line our grocery shelves and pantries. They may be very harmful, especially to children. FD&C Yellow No. 5 (tartrazine) is one of the most widely used food dyes and is known to contribute to asthma attacks, hives, and other allergic reactions. This coloring is found in cereals, baked goods, snack foods, candies, and beverages.

The Feingold Hypothesis, proffered through the research of Dr. Benjamin Feingold, postulates that food additives may cause hyperactivity and inattention in children. His research revealed that as many as 40 to 50 percent of children are sensitive to preservatives, artificial colors, and food dyes. There are many natural sweeteners and preservatives available that can meet the same intended purpose. Again, reading your food labels will help you cut down on these useless and likely harmful ingredients. Examples of acceptable natural preservatives and colorings include ascorbic acid, soy and sunflower lecithins, beet juice, cardamom, and turmeric.

HOW OUR CELLS ARE AFFECTED BY THE FOODS WE EAT

Proper cellular function is the difference between health and disease. And what we eat affects the quality of our cells and how well they function.

The *cell*, from the Latin root cella, meaning "small room," is the basic structural, functional, and biological unit of all known living organisms. The three major cell components include the cell membrane, the nucleus with DNA, and the mitochondria.

The *cell membrane* is the outside of the cell and is made up of fats—specifically, the types of fats we eat. A healthy cell membrane is selectively permeable and smart, taking in nutrients and oxygen from our bloodstream that are provided by the foods we eat and rejecting circulating toxins that try to penetrate its barrier.

The quality of our cell membranes are impacted by the types of fats we have consumed over the prior few months. Healthy fats, like omega-3s from fish and certain nuts and seeds, support a healthy cell membrane. The **Wildatarian** lifestyle supports the assimilation of healthy fats to the cell membrane through rich omega-3 fatty acids and conjugated linolenic acid found in lamb, or from other healthy fats of avocado and seeds. Even **WF-Wildatarian** types can consume seeds and other more easily digested healthy fats. Conversely, a Standard American Diet of fast food, pastries, and packaged foods that contain hydrogenated fats make the cell membrane brittle and vulnerable to the entry of toxins that can affect the DNA.

DNA is found in the core or nucleus of the cell. This is where the complete set of genes or genetic material—the genome—is located. According to Bruce Ames, PhD, a scientist at the University of California Berkeley, each of us encounters from 1,000 to 10,000 potential injuries to the integrity of our DNA daily ... meaning the integrity of our cells and our DNA is under constant attack! Fortunately, the DNA repair mechanisms, along with healthy cell membranes and a healthy immune system, keep the potential damage to our genes under control. However, when cell integrity is compromised, the cell membrane becomes less selective, and damaging toxins like fat-soluble pesticides penetrate the cell membrane at higher rates and reach the DNA. Here is where unfavorable gene expression can occur. Just like a light switch, the wrong genes are turned on and the right genes are turned off, negatively impacting our health.

Damage to the DNA can also occur from compounds called reactive oxygen species (or ROS), also known as free radicals. ROS substances are like trash—they are generated as part of our body's normal processes or as toxic byproducts of unhealthy reactions in the body. Antioxidants are like a Pac-Man to the trash, eating up those free radicals. We take in antioxidants from eating clean, whole, **Wildatarian** foods.

Mitochondria are the powerhouses of the cell. Here, energy is produced from the nutrients in food. These energy converters help you move, think, and function. The mitochondria use fats and glucose to produce this energy. Oxygen-rich food such as leafy greens, which provide chlorophyll and iron, also support mitochondrial function.

In the 1988 Surgeon General's Report on Nutrition and Health, former Surgeon General Dr. C. Everett Koop wrote:

> *Food sustains us, ... Yet what we eat may affect our risk for several of the leading causes of death for Americans, notably, coronary heart disease, stroke, arteriosclerosis, diabetes, and some types of cancer. These disorders together now account for more than two-thirds of all deaths in the United States. ... enough has been learned about the overall health impact of the dietary patterns now prevalent in our society to recommend significant changes in those patterns.*

Nearly thirty years later, our commercial food supply still contributes to disease. It is up to each one of us to make wise choices when selecting what we put into our bodies. It is not about depriving ourselves of the foods we love—it is about making better choices for ourselves and for our families with ingredients that taste great and nourish the body. Eating well is not about a state of deprivation; instead, it's about making informed lifestyle choices that promote health and wellness. Love and nourish your cells, and they will love and nourish you back.

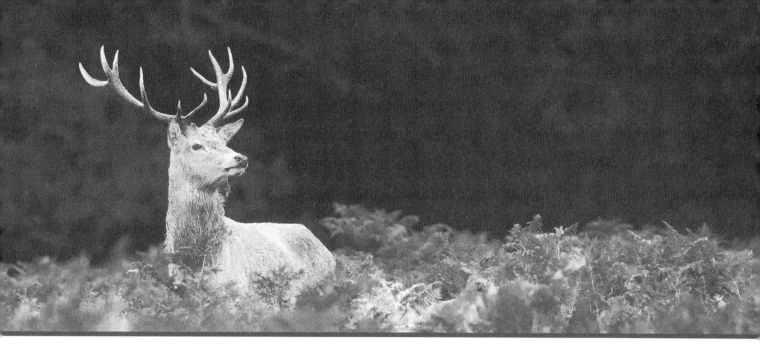

CHAPTER 5

THE WILDATARIAN APPROACH: PROTECTIVE PROTEINS

The almighty protein is the microscopic machine that drives life and helps to make muscles, tissue, skin, enzymes, and hormones. It provides us with the essential amino acids (the building blocks of proteins) that our bodies need but cannot produce; they must be consumed. The proteins we ingest from eating animal products contain all nine essential amino acids, while most plant-based proteins alone do not and must be paired with other complementary amino acid food sources to complete the amino acid picture. Those nine essential amino acids are:

- histidine
- isoleucine
- leucine
- lysine
- methionine
- phenylalanine
- threonine
- tryptophan
- valine

As I've mentioned in previous chapters, consuming the meat from commercially raised animals may be hurting us. Consuming these meats may change how our bodies manage amyloids. The inhumane living conditions for our factory-farmed meat and poultry coupled with the food they are fed may promote amyloid fibrils in these animals. Interestingly, a study out of Michigan

State University found that when healthy ducks were put in crowded pens, 71 percent of them developed amyloidosis (a disease condition associated with amyloids). In the most crowded pens, spontaneous deaths from amyloidosis began at six months of age.

When we eat these meats and poultry, their imbalances are passed on to us, and these harmful protein fragments can attach themselves to our organs and tissues and may eventually lead to the buildup of plaque-like deposits, especially as our bodies become compromised by age, stress, inflammation and as our quality-control mechanisms (such as cell repair) decline. These amyloids are not destroyed, even when the animal's meat is cooked at high temperatures, and, consequently, our food goes from nourishing to devastating.

Researchers at the University of Cambridge credit the explosion of interest in amyloids to the fact that many of the disorders associated with amyloids are no longer rare, *and amyloids contribute to the most common and debilitating medical conditions in the modern world.* Amyloids have now been implicated in approximately fifty major disorders, including Alzheimer's, Parkinson's, autoimmune diseases, and Type 2 diabetes. They may manifest in symptoms such as seizures, tremors, migraines, and debilitating fatigue.

The aim of the **Wildatarian** diet is to reduce dietary amyloids likely found in most inflamed animals.

THE PERILS OF AMERICAN MEAT

The stressful conditions that animals bred for food live in have been linked with chronic inflammation in their tissues. Cows are treated with repeated rounds of hormones and antibiotics and are fed a grain-based diet that their bodies cannot break down. This shifts their otherwise-neutral stomach pH toward acidity, lowers their immune function, and promotes illness and disease, which necessitates the constant dosing of antibiotics.

Commercially raised beef also contains a less-healthy type of fat, primarily omega-6, and virtually no beneficial omega-3 fatty acids. Omega-6 fatty acids, while essential, can contribute to inflammation when present in high amounts, especially in relation to the omega-3s. In addition to antibiotics, commercial cow meat contains xenoestrogens—industrially made compounds that mimic the hormone estrogen and which are stored in the animal's fatty tissue.

Sources of xenoestrogens include pesticides and growth hormones, both of which are given to cattle. Domesticated animals bred for consumption, typically contain much higher overall fat content. Therefore, these higher-fat animals may store higher levels of xenoestrogens than their wild cousins. When we eat this meat, these hormone disruptors are then stored in our fatty tissue. The more fatty tissue we store, the more of this toxin we store. Xenoestrogens are now suspected to be linked to many health issues, including uterine fibroids, PCOS, menstrual irregularities, and even hormonal cancers.

Commercially raised poultry is just as problematic. Chickens are raised in inhumane conditions, stuck in tight-fitting cages for most of their lives. They are fed a pesticide- and herbicide-laden diet full of soy and other foods incompatible with their digestion and are given a variety of medications designed to improve feed utilization and accelerate growth. Antibiotics also may be given to prevent disease and shorten time to market.

Food can be our medicine, but the wrong food is contributing to the ever-growing abundance of resistant bacterial and viral strains. Through daily consumption of domesticated animal products, we are feeding the creation of a disease state. Through clinical outcomes in our practice, we have witnessed that when we stop feeding the body with amyloid-producing substances and support the **HealAndSeal** approach, balance in the body is restored.

WILDATARIAN MEAT CHOICES

Thousands of years ago, domesticated animals did not exist. Animals were cultivated and hunted in their natural habitats. Wild game *is* the original grass-fed, free-range, sustainable meat source. Once exclusive to hunters, wild game meats are becoming ever more popular in American cuisine, and we believe eating these supports lower oxidative stress in our bodies.

Most wild game is generally leaner, relatively higher in omega-3 fatty acids, and often lower in cholesterol (due to the low saturated fat content). These meats are not tainted by steroids, antibiotics, and other additives. Additionally, wild game is richer in minerals, especially zinc and iron, which are necessary for bone, brain, and gut health.

These more desirable traits are due to their natural wild vegetation diet as opposed to the grain and corn fed to their domesticated counterparts. I call buffalo and bison "the skinny cow," because this meat contains up to 70 percent less fat, half the cholesterol, and higher iron stores than beef. Our iron stores are often depleted, especially in cases of pathogenic infections like staph and candida. This is often exacerbated by eating a diet full of high-sugar and high-amyloid foods.

The dishes we feature in our recipes include wild meat such as buffalo, bison, duck, elk, venison, wild boar, lamb, and Cornish game hen. (Although lamb and Cornish game hen are not wild, we include them as acceptable substitutes). These meats have rich and complex flavors that add new dimensions to your cooking. If you are a **WF–Wildatarian** type, then you will avoid the higher-fat **Wildatarian** meats such as lamb, Cornish game hen and duck during the **Rebalance** phase.

> Wild meat is prepared in a similar manner to traditional cuts of meat. A slow cooker or a pressure cooker are essential kitchen helpers to ensure a juicy, tender, and tasty result. Using a hot cast iron skillet and cooking with a searing method also works well.
>
> Roasting duck, pheasant, or goose is similar to cooking chicken or turkey. I use a Le Creuset Dutch oven for roasting. Preheat the oven to 400 degrees, season the bird, and let the Dutch oven do the rest. The recipes provide specific instructions.

If you are going to eat potentially higher amyloid-containing meats such as beef or chicken, you should choose organic and/or pasture-fed, and make sure they come from a reliable source. Although pasture-fed is definitely better than commercially raised animal meat and fowl, it doesn't mean these types of animals are raised without "extras," such as pesticides, hormones, antibiotics, and other toxins. In addition, U.S. Food and Drug Administration (FDA) regulations regarding terms like pasture fed, grass fed, pasture raised, cage free, free range and grass finished are confusing and poorly enforced.

These definitions are tricky. For example, to meet the standard for the FDA's *free range* designation, "producers must demonstrate to the Agency that the poultry has been allowed access to the outside"; the chickens can be caged again for the night. "Outside" could be a gorgeous pasture of rolling hills, as is in the case of Polyface Farms, a top quality chicken vendor in Virginia. Or outside could be a paved parking lot in the middle of a polluted area. Some producers include a fenced-in section of open concrete in their grow-out houses, with enough room for maybe 5 percent of the thousands of chickens in that house, and this may technically satisfy the FDA definition.

Keep in mind that if commercial agriculture practices start being applied to our wild animals, then they likely will become susceptible to inflammation and disease and ultimately will become unhealthy food choices as well. So visit your local farmer and encourage sustainable, wild practices for our livestock. Use the power of the dollar! Get to know the person who is selling you your meat—your health will be better for it. Practice the tenets of a **Wildatarian** lifestyle and only purchase sustainably and wild raised animals, dairy, fish and shellfish.

WILDATARIAN EGG CHOICES

Choose eggs from organic and free-range birds—they are richer in good, essential fatty acids. Through our practice, we have found that duck eggs may be more easily digestible, especially for those with sulfur sensitivities. All yolks, however, are sulfur-rich food sources, so don't overdo it if you are a **WS–** or **WFS–Wildatarian** type, and completely avoid yolks during your Rebalance phase. As an added note, even with a sulfur sensitivity, I still allow whole eggs in baked goods or as a minor ingredient in recipes.

WILDATARIAN FISH CHOICES

Farm-raised fish are not recommended on the **Wildatarian** diet due to the many unhealthy substances they are exposed to during farming.

PESTICIDES: Fish farmers have been using pesticides in an attempt to kill sea lice, a common problem when farming fish. These pesticides accumulate in the tissue of farmed fish, circulate in the ocean, and concentrate in the fat of wild marine life.

ANTIBIOTICS: As with land animals, farm-raised fish often are given antibiotics in an effort to stave off disease. These diseases come as a result of their living conditions and the crowded way in which they are kept.

DIOXINS/PCBS: Dioxins and PCBs are toxins known to impair the human reproductive, immune, endocrine, and nervous systems. Dioxins tend to be high in farmed fish.

CANTHAXANTHIN: This is a synthetic pigment that gives farm-raised salmon its pink color. Wild salmon eat marine life such as shrimp and krill, providing carotenoids that give the wild fish its natural rich pink color. Farmed salmon is raised in confined tanks or underwater net pens, and often fed food that is unnatural to its digestion, such as corn. As a result, farmed salmon has to be "food-colored" to achieve the pigment the consumer expects. Canthaxanthin has been banned in the United Kingdom.

There is one exception to my "no farmed fish" rule. Some retailers, such as Whole Foods, are creating their own fish farming operations in order to meet high demand. Get to know your Whole Foods fish salesperson; ask them about their farms and find out if their practices meet your discerning standards. If they do, you can go ahead and purchase their products without concern. Please recheck often, as economic considerations often drive retailers to change practices.

My seafood recipes include primarily those wild fish listed as low on the bio-accumulation[4] list. I recommend avoiding larger fish like tuna (although skipjack, a smaller tuna, can be used), grouper, orange roughy, swordfish, and tilefish, especially for pregnant or nursing women. Choose fish that come from cleaner waters, and avoid those that come from highly polluted areas. Most white fish is otherwise a very lean protein source, rich in the good omega-3 fatty acids, easily digestible, and simple to prepare. I always had a fear of cooking fish before I realized how easy it is. Now, I cook fish when time is scarce. Eating fish at least once a week is a good goal, and my recipes make it an easy one to achieve. Most fish recipes provided in this book take under fifteen minutes to prepare. Some of my favorite fish include flounder, snapper, and

---

4   Bio-accumulation is the increase in concentration of a substance (in this case mercury or other heavy metals) as it moves up the food chain.

salmon. (Salmon, trout, and sea bass are not suitable for the **Rebalance** phase of your plan if you are a **WF–** or **WFS–Wildatarian** type).

WILDATARIAN PLANT-BASED PROTEINS

Plant-based proteins include sources from beans, legumes, nuts, seeds, and grains. I include certain beans and legumes in my **Wildatarian** approach. The preferred choices are the varieties lower in starch and mycotoxins, such as chickpeas and black, red, pinto, and kidney beans. If you have dysbiosis or candida or have recurrent strep infections, then avoid green and split peas, green beans, and pea protein. The suggested beans and legumes are wild by their very nature. They are a rich source of vitamins and minerals necessary for cellular function and constitute a sustainable, plant-based protein source that is virtually unchanged from how nature created it.

BEANS AND LEGUMES

Beans may have a beneficial effect on our microbiome. Unfavorable alterations in our microbiome—the totality of bacteria living in various organs of our body—have been linked to a host of conditions, such as autoimmunity, autism, mental health disorders, and Type 2 diabetes. Various species of bacteria make up this system, and they need good food to survive and thrive. Beans, with their high fiber content, are some of the most favorable foods that allow the biome to function at an optimum level. In particular, chickpeas (also called garbanzo beans) serve as food for the beneficial bacteria in our gut. I consider them to be one of the healthiest beans for the gut biome.

I do recommend staying away from all beans, even the healthiest ones, if you've been diagnosed with significant candida or small intestinal bacterial overgrowth (SIBO), because they may contribute to feeding the wrong bacteria in your gut. Someone with ulcerative colitis will also need to be careful with beans. If you eat beans and experience unpleasant symptoms such as pain, gas, or bloat, cut back on the serving size or discontinue completely until symptoms resolve. You may also try pureeing the beans to help with digestibility, because this process breaks down their insoluble fiber skins. Some bean varieties contain high oxalate levels. Please refer to the oxalate discussion later in this chapter to see if you need to avoid certain beans.

THE ROLE OF BEANS IN BALANCING CHRONIC DISEASE

Beans are tiny but mighty soldiers that wage the war on chronic disease. One cup of beans contains roughly fifteen grams of fiber, which is approximately half of the recommended dietary allowance. That fiber is vitally important to your overall health, because it helps regulate cholesterol, blood sugar, and weight.

In the battle to lower cholesterol, oatmeal is not your only friend. The soluble fiber in beans helps to lower cholesterol by creating a gel-like substance in the digestive tract that helps to reduce the absorption of unwanted cholesterol by the intestines.

Fiber is also a winner for keeping you full longer. The soluble fiber in beans also helps stabilize blood sugar levels after a meal, because it slows the conversion of carbohydrates to sugar in our systems. This stabilization is important for those with diabetes, insulin resistance, and hypoglycemia. By staying full longer, we are less apt to reach for snack and junk foods that can contribute to weight gain and blood sugar dysregulation.

In addition to managing cholesterol, blood sugar, and weight, beans also top the USDA's list of twenty high-antioxidant sources of common foods. A study was conducted on more than 100 different fruits, vegetables, and berries. Various beans held four coveted spots on this list. Red beans were in the number one spot, beating out wild blueberries as the food with the highest concentration of antioxidants per serving. Pinto and kidney beans rounded the top four. Remember that antioxidants are so important to good health, because they fight the free radicals that are produced as part of our normal metabolism when we consume inflammatory foods or when we engage in unhealthy lifestyle practices.

Beans work exceedingly well for creating convertible dishes. My family incorporates beans into our daily fare. A pot of beans can be transformed into an elegant puréed soup, a Mexican-style salsa, a dip, a spread for sandwiches, or even a side for eggs. They are a great ingredient for a casserole dish or a cold or warm salad, and are easy to drop into soups.

In this book, I share my family's *Cuban Black Beans* recipe with you. This recipe is so versatile that it can also be used to create multiple other meals with my convertible options.

Chickpeas are a favorite in *Wild Game Chili* as well as for the *Mediterranean-Style Quinoa Salad*. Kidney and pinto beans are perfect for the *Red Beans and Rice* recipe. I prepare lentils very simply with sweet root vegetables.

Two added benefits to cooking with beans are that they keep nicely in the refrigerator and their flavors intensify with time. However, a good rule of thumb is to use the beans within four days of cooking. The use of garlic, lemon, or apple cider vinegar in bean dishes helps to preserve the beans so they don't get moldy too quickly. But remember, garlic is a high sulfur compound, so skip the garlic if it's not part of your **Wildatarian** type.

DRIED OR CANNED?

As to the big question of dried or canned, I like to use dried beans when I am making a big batch to use for multiple meals. I think the flavor of dried beans is better, and one sixteen-ounce bag will yield five to six cups of cooked beans, or about eight servings. Talk about economical—a bag of dried beans usually costs less than two dollars. This can be helpful for families going **Wildatarian** on a budget.

Dried beans require soaking (unless you own a pressure cooker). Most of my bean recipes call for a pressure cooker. You can use a large Dutch oven or slow cooker instead, but I believe the time savings and flavor benefits from a pressure cooker are worth the investment. Some people are afraid to experiment with this appliance, but I assure you that today's models are safe and easy to use. The great thing about a pressure cooker is that once it becomes pressurized, you just turn down the heat and the pressure cooker does the rest. When the cooker is depressurized, open the lid, add additional ingredients as specified, and let the beans cook down to the desired consistency.

> My pressure cooker has been a saving grace for me with foods that would otherwise take hours and hours to prepare. This appliance was a hand-me-down from my mom and is over thirty years old; I use it regularly. Beans are my go-to meal when I have a busy day ahead; a pressure cooker can cut cooking time in half. When I get up, I put the beans in the pressure cooker with water, onion, and salt. By the time I am ready for work, the beans are cooked, so when my day is finished, they just need to be warmed and thickened. Sometimes, I even cook them the evening before instead.

Canned beans such as black, pinto, cannellini, or chickpeas are a good choice for dips and salsas, or in a pinch when time is really scarce. Rinse and drain canned beans, and lay them atop a gluten-free whole grain tortilla or a mound of fresh or sautéed greens.

If you are going to use canned beans, please ensure the cans are BPA-free. BPA is an industrial chemical that has been used to make certain plastics and resins since the 1960s. Many brands also are now offering beans in paper boxes and glass jars.

SOY

Soy is a source of phytoestrogens that can help manage menopausal symptoms, and it is an alternative for anyone sensitive to cow dairy.

Soy is the number two crop grown in the United States (corn is number one). It is fed to cattle, chickens, and pigs. It is used as a filler in foods such as burgers, ketchup, and cereal. Soybean oil is used for frying many products from fish sticks to chips. This means that without realizing it, most of us are consuming more soy than we think.

Unless otherwise specified on the label, most of the soy used in food products has been genetically modified. Soy is included in a group of foods called goitrogens, which can promote the formation of a goiter (an enlarged thyroid) and may disrupt thyroid function. Additionally, soy can bind to zinc, a mineral important in thyroid function, immune health, and glucose metabolism, thus making zinc less available to the body. The keys are to consume organic as much as possible and to be watchful of how much you are taking in. Do not consume soy daily.

HEART-HEALTHY WILDATARIAN NUT CHOICES

Nuts are another great source of plant-based protein. While it is true that nuts have been traditionally thought of as a high-fat food, **Wildatarian**-friendly nut choices contain heart-protective fats to support healthy cholesterol and blood sugar levels. They are rich in both nutrients and health-promoting phytochemicals. Many nuts are a great source of B vitamins, minerals, vitamin E, calcium, and essential fatty acids, including omega-3. Unless you are sensitive to nuts or have fat malabsroption, daily consumption of various types of nuts can confer many health benefits without adding pounds.

AVOIDING CERTAIN NUTS AND LEGUMES IS PART OF THE WILDATARIAN APPROACH

Certain types of nuts and legumes, such as peanuts, peas, green beans, Brazil nuts, and sesame seeds tend to be high in mycotoxins, which may force the body to deal with an increased burden of mold. According to a Food and Agriculture Organization (FAO) study, approximately 25 percent of the global food and feed crop output is affected by mycotoxins, which may feed unwanted pathogens, disrupt the integrity and balance of the gut biome, and promote amyloid formation.

NUTS. My simple recommendation is to consume small amounts of nuts daily. If you are a **WF–** or **WFS–Wildatarian** type, then you will avoid all nuts during the Rebalance phase, although some nuts (such as almonds, hazelnuts, and walnuts) will be allowed in the long term. If your type allows fats, then just a handful of almonds, walnuts, cashews, hazelnuts, or pecans—approximately ten to fifteen—will give you the benefits without excessive calories. For nut butters, I prefer cashew and almond.

SEEDS. If you are a **WF–** or **WFS–Wildatarian** type, then seeds—such as chia, pumpkin, sunflower, and flax—are generally easier for your body to break down, For the **WF–** and **WFS–**

Wildatarian type, your seed butter of choice should be sunflower butter. The **HealAndSeal** program provides specific details.

Like nuts, seeds should be a vital part of our diet. These seeds can be incorporated into meals, snacks, and desserts. Chia seeds in particular are high in iron, folate, calcium, magnesium, omega-3 fatty acids, and soluble fiber. This super seed's calcium and magnesium promote bone and dental health, while the omega-3s help your heart by lowering triglycerides (the fats in your blood that when in excess can cause heart disease). Seeds should be kept in the refrigerator or in an airtight container away from light.

Purchase nuts and seeds in raw form when available; they contain more of the beneficial essential fatty acids. Raw nuts may be less digestible, so we recommend soaking them overnight in salt water. Place raw nuts in a glass container with a small amount of water and sea salt. In the morning, dehydrate them in the oven at the lowest possible temperature until they become crisp. We don't recommend sprouting, which is a three-day process and may confer some mold. Again, mold is anti-**Wildatarian**.

Avoid commercially roasted nuts, because they are typically prepared at high temperatures—a process where healthy oils can convert to trans-fats, become hydrogenated, and cause the production of free radicals. These can promote the buildup of plaque in your arteries and increase overall inflammation. In addition, heavier nuts such as cashew and Brazil may not be for you. Seeds such as pumpkin and sunflower may be a better option.

COCONUTS

Both coconut milk and shredded coconut can be used for cooking and baking. Coconut milk is made from coconut pulp and water, but the milk varies in creaminess depending on the brand. Coconut milk is available whole in cans, or diluted in cardboard or plastic beverage containers. I always opt for the unsweetened varieties. **WF–Wildatarian**s should avoid full-fat coconut milk and instead opt for the coconut milk beverage.

Coconut may be protective to the thyroid gland. It contains lauric acid, which has antimicrobial, antiviral, and antifungal properties. Although canned coconut milk is high in fat, the fat consists of short-chain and medium-chain fatty acids that the body quickly turns into energy. For some, coconut may actually aid in weight loss. When buying coconut milk beverage or any other dairy-free milk alternative, please choose one without carrageenan[5] and with as few ingredients as possible. Coconut is considered rich in oxalates.

OXALATES

Some varieties of legumes, vegetables, and nuts have a high oxalate content. Oxalate metabolism impairment has been linked to mental health issues, including anxiety, depression, and even mania. For some individuals, excess oxalates can result in joint pain, kidney stones, gallstones, chronic fatigue, mental health issues, and even contribute to autism.

Unfortunately, because of differences in farming practices, specific food varieties, and cooking techniques, there is no full agreement on what constitutes a high-oxalate food, although peanuts appear on most oxalate avoidance lists. Through our clinical outcomes, we have established that black beans have higher levels of oxalates, as do almonds and coconut.

If you have one of the conditions above, please talk to your doctor and follow a low-oxalate diet. In addition, some medicines may contain oxalates, and you should consult with your doctor regarding this. In general, if arabinose[6] is present, oxalate avoidance is recommended. We advise our clients to avoid:

- coconut
- almonds
- peanuts
- beets

- spinach
- swiss chard
- okra
- black beans

- parsley
- quinoa
- oats

Remember, the almighty protein drives life and serves as the building block for healthy muscles, tissue, skin, enzymes, neurotransmitters, and even hormones. Make your protein choices wisely, and promote healthy habits by following our **Wildatarian** approach and lifestyle.

---

5   Carrageenan is an additive that can cause inflammation and gut irritation. It is widely used in processed foods for its gelling, thickening, and stabilizing properties.

6   Arabinose is a metabolite of candida, a fungus that can cause a variety of symptoms if overgrown in the body.

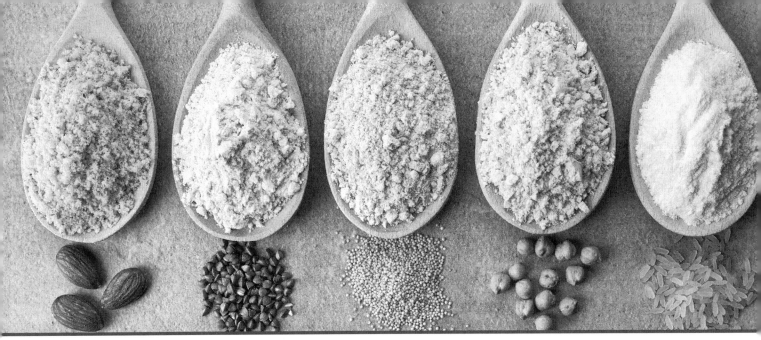

CHAPTER 6

WILDATARIAN GRAINS

Humans have been eating whole grains for thousands of years. Rich in fiber, antioxidants, B vitamins, and minerals, whole grains have played a crucial role in the rise and prosperity of civilization. But somehow, society has lost its way, stripping these grains through commonplace food production practices and leaving them as nutrient-poor starches. In my recipes, I use ancient as well as newly recognized whole grains, which will help us reconnect with the food of our ancestors and move toward the modern **Wildatarian** approach and lifestyle.

What exactly is a whole grain? Well, it is just as the name implies. It is "whole," meaning that both the inner kernel (germ) and the outer husk of the grain (bran) are present, which preserves all the natural nutrients and minerals. Ironically, before the invention of the steel roller, only the wealthy were able to afford low-nutrient milled and refined grains. However, this invention in the late 1800s made the production of refined grains more efficient and less expensive, making them more accessible to all socioeconomic classes. Refined flours quickly became popular and prevalent as they were praised for their extended shelf life and fluffy, light quality when used in baking. This initiated the mass production of nutrient-poor flours—a refinement revolution.

Refinement removes the majority of a grain's nutrients and fiber—the elements of grain that help to stabilize blood-sugar levels, support good cholesterol, and promote cellular health. The remaining white starch has minimal nutrient content and does little more than raise blood sugar levels and convert into fatty tissue if not burned as fuel by the body.

Sometimes refined grains are labeled as "enriched" when nutrients are added to the flour. This is ironic: refined grain manufacturers attempt to replace the nutrients they removed during the refining process. The body, however, does not break down these enriched flours in the same way it does the original whole grain. The minerals and vitamins have properties that allow them to function synergistically when paired together, as they are in whole grains. These synergistic relationships ultimately provide the body with greater benefits than those included in enriched products. For example, the interaction of magnesium and B vitamins found in whole grains helps to better manage stress levels, a phenomenon which may not occur at all when metabolized separately or when using synthetic forms of these vitamins and minerals.

Depending on your genetic makeup, you may or may not be able to properly metabolize your B vitamins. For example, if you have one of the many MTHFR (methylenetetrahydrofolate reductase) gene mutations, you may not be able to convert folate (vitamin B9) into its active form needed for many key processes in the body. This is the problem of inefficient methylation. Unfortunately, refined grains and products made from their flours, are enriched with folic acid—a form of vitamin B9 that those with inefficient methylation genetics will not be able to use and in fact may be harmed by it. Eating grains in their natural form eliminates this problem.

My **Wildatarian** approach does not eliminate all grains. Instead, the lifestyle excludes those grains that are not ancient and/or have relatively high glycemic indexes, and those that contain pesticides and chemicals that disrupt the biome of the body's digestive tract. Our **Wildatarian** grains are nutrient-rich rather than metabolically disruptive.

GLUTEN AND GLYPHOSATES

You may notice that many of the non-**Wildatarian** grains contain gluten. In the past decade, gluten, in particular, has emerged as one of the most controversial topics in the conversation about modern health. Gluten is a protein found most abundantly in wheat and its many varieties, while also making up a percentage of the chemical compositions of rye, barley, spelt, and kamut.

Gluten-containing foods made in the United States have unfortunately become indigestible for a large percentage of the population. We do not see the same high levels of gluten intolerance in countries such as France and Italy that we see in the United States. In fact, many of my clients who are sensitive to gluten in the United States do very well when eating gluten in those countries. Studies show that the standard wheat grown in the United States can be highly inflammatory, because it is highly hybridized and sprayed with dangerous herbicides.

GLYPHOSATE, GLUTEN INTOLERANCE, AND METHYLATION

Why is gluten such an indigestible protein? My hypothesis is that the combination of hybridization practices (where wheat varieties are bred to contain unrecognizable gluten proteins) and the use of glyphosate is a contributing factor to gluten/glyphosate-induced leaky gut epidemic. According to a theory postulated by Stephanie Seneff, PhD (a senior research scientist at Massachusetts Institute of Technology) and one to which I subscribe, glyphosate contamination in gluten makes proteins (both plant and animal based) more difficult to break down. Glyphosate is routinely sprayed on gluten-containing crops and is the active ingredient in the herbicide Roundup—a substance used pervasively in commercial agriculture. Unfortunately, glyphosates disrupt the pancreatic enzymes that metabolize proteins.

Dr. Seneff also co-authored a paper with Anthony Samsel showing how glyphosate mimics glycine—one of the most prevalent of the amino acids that form the basic building blocks of life and a key player in our methylation pathways. Glycine is necessary for protein digestion. When the body believes it is already producing glycine because it is tricked by the glyphosate, it stops producing the real glycine, impairing our ability to properly methylate and digest protein.

Other important methylation pathways and their mechanisms in our bodies can be disrupted through this mechanism. These include hormone balance, fat metabolism, cholesterol metabolism, and the carrying of our neurotransmitters across our blood-brain barrier so we can use them for sleep and mood regulation.

Glyphosate is a destructive herbicide on so many levels. It has been implicated in Alzheimer's, Parkinson's, depression, and cancer. As an aside, the state of California has officially designated glyphosate as cancer causing, requiring warning labels on all products that contain it. In addition, the World Health Organization has designated glyphosate a "probable carcinogen." France has just passed a law mandating the removal of this chemical from their agriculture within the next several years.

I had the opportunity to discuss this phenomenon personally with Dr. Seneff. Along with illuminating how glyphosates affect our ability to properly digest protein (plant- and animal-based), our discussion focused on how glyphosates may impair our body's ability to properly process sulfur. We hypothesize that sulfur-processing mechanisms are becoming less efficient, because glyphosate impairs our body's ability to convert sulfur to sulfate, the form of sulfur we use to make tendons and ligaments and that helps to process hormones and neurotransmitters. This is contributing to what I believe to be a growing epidemic of sulfur intolerance.

Sulfur is necessary for mental health, endocrine health, collagen structure matrix, and detoxification. Sulfur is also important for digestive health. Impaired sulfur processing capabilities have been implicated in Crohn's disease, ulcerative colitis, irritable bowel syndrome and even celiac disease. It has also been linked to rheumatoid arthritis. Individuals with the CBS, SUOX and BH4 gene polymorphisms are further at risk of being predisposed to the above conditions when these genes are expressed.

SHORTCOMINGS OF TODAY'S GLUTEN-FREE WAVE

As a result of this gluten intolerance epidemic, gluten-free (GF) eating is becoming a ubiquitous trend. However, most GF products are made with white rice, corn, sorghum, and potatoes—ingredients that, when commonly consumed, can contribute to metabolic dysfunction, especially when combined in one product. Individually, these ingredients can be acceptable if they are organic, non-GMO, and paired with high protein **Wildatarian** grains. However, when combined, they only offer refined carbohydrate content and low nutrient value, making them a diabetes time bomb. Remember that according to the USDA, 88 percent of corn is genetically modified. These crops are typically sprayed with Roundup to limit pests, which continues the glyphosate nightmare.

READING LABELS IS KEY

When determining which grains to use, reading food labels is imperative. Labeling for oats, wheat, and other grains must state stone ground, rolled, steel cut, or 100-percent whole grain. Note that because quinoa and other alternative grains such as buckwheat, amaranth, and millet are not typically refined, they may not have this specific labeling. If the label says a flour is enriched or unbleached, then it is not made from whole grain.

WILDATARIAN WHOLE GRAINS

The whole grains I recommend and use in my recipes are some of my personal favorites like quinoa, brown rice, oats, and buckwheat. Other whole grains not specifically featured include teff, amaranth, and millet. I usually cook up to three days' worth of quinoa and steel cut oats at one time. This is an efficient way to get your fill of these "good-for-us" grains without spending hours in the kitchen. Don't make more than three to four days' worth, though, or they may start fermenting in your refrigerator—possibly impacting your digestive system in undesirable ways.

QUINOA has become one of my favorite high-protein grains. It along with buckwheat has the highest protein content of all of the grains and is a complete protein—one that provides all of the essential amino acids. Quinoa is GF, tends to be lower in allergens, and is very versatile. In terms of its consistency, I consider quinoa to be a cross between couscous and grits. Quinoa has a nutty flavor and cooks in fifteen minutes.

When preparing quinoa, first soak and rinse the seeds in water. I use a mesh colander so none of the tiny seeds escape down the kitchen sink drain. Rinsing aids digestion, because it removes the bitter saponins that coat the seeds. Although categorized as a grain, quinoa is actually the seed of a leafy plant that is a distant cousin of beets and spinach and, therefore, has oxalate properties. Please refer to the oxalate discussion in Chapter 5 to see if you should be avoiding these foods. Remember that there is no one healthy food for everyone; we are all bio-individual.

Try quinoa for breakfast in *Quinoa with Cinnamon, Apples, and Walnuts*. Serve it as a cold salad with *Mediterranean-Style Quinoa Salad* or as a warm side dish. Mix it with any vegetable, cheese, or fruit and nut for a hearty and nutritious meal. Quinoa is being used in many GF pasta varieties, and is preferable to GF pastas made from white rice or corn flour.

BROWN RICE is another great high-protein grain that provides many recipe options. Brown rice combined with beans creates a complete protein. It is no wonder rice and beans has been a staple meal in many parts of the world for centuries.

The rice bran found in brown rice also contains gamma-oryzanol, a compound that has a cholesterol-lowering effect. It also contains B vitamins and minerals important for balancing blood sugar and adrenal function.

Brown rice is chewier, nuttier, and richer in nutrients than traditional white rice. It can be used as a main dish, side, or dessert, or even for breakfast. Brown rice comes in short, medium, and long grain, as well as in basmati and jasmine varieties. Note that in both *Duck Paella* and *Coconut Arroz con Leche*, I use short-grain brown rice instead of traditional white arborio.

Brown rice pasta is a perfectly delicious and GF noodle alternative that holds up nicely in soups and main courses. If cooked incorrectly, however, you may be left with a lumpy, gummy heap. The trick to avoiding this mess is to add one tablespoon of olive oil to the water before boiling. While the pasta is cooking, take a fork and carefully separate the strands. When the pasta becomes al dente, drain it in a colander and rinse it well with warm water. Then, combine the pasta with a teaspoon of olive oil in a large bowl. This will help keep the pasta from sticking together. The brown rice/quinoa pasta combination is my favorite.

OATS are known for their high-fiber content and also for selenium, a potent antioxidant. Additionally, they are a good source of polyunsaturated fats. They are the go-to grain for lowering cholesterol and stabilizing blood-sugar levels. Because oats are insoluble, they are not included in the **Rebalance** phase of any **Wildatarian** type; they may be difficult on the lower colon as we move to **HealAndSeal** your gut.

Oat flour is versatile in GF baking and makes great pancakes, breads, and muffins. When cooking with oats, I only use rolled or steel-cut varieties. Both are nutritionally sound, though I prefer the steel-cut type due to its tendency to hold up well in the refrigerator. The wonderful thing about oats is they are easy to infuse with flavors of your choice. When you pair them with fruit, as in *Berryful Steel-Cut Oatmeal*, the oats carry the berry flavors, which are further infused over time, so this is an ideal choice to make ahead.

It is extremely important to read food labels when choosing oatmeal. Some oatmeal varieties, especially those packaged in serving-size bags, are loaded with preservatives and high fructose corn syrup that undermine the health benefits of the oats. Again, as a bio-individual reminder, oats are a moderately high-oxalate food, so avoid if you are following a low-oxalate plan.

BUCKWHEAT is another ancient and GF grain-like seed that is also a complete protein that has a high fiber content. Buckwheat flour is good for combining with other GF varieties like quinoa and chickpea flours. Delicious breakfast options that use buckwheat flour include *Banana, Buckwheat, and Chocolate Chip Muffins* and *Pumpkin Buckwheat Crepes*. Beware that buckwheat flour can make your food look almost purple—don't worry, it's the great polyphenols that give the grain this odd color.

GRAIN GOODNESS

Grains are essential for minerals, vitamins, proteins, fiber and digestion. Now more than ever, we must vote with our food dollars. Genetically modified grains and herbicide-sprayed gluten are contributing to impaired protein and sulfur mechanisms, with devastating downstream impacts.

Getting the goodness of grains from **Wildatarian** varieties is easy. This book offers many ways to enjoy them. These **Wildatarian** grains contain from two to six grams of fiber per serving. Thirty-five grams of fiber per day is a great and realistic goal you can achieve for yourself with the proper awareness and when using simple, ancient-grain substitutions. Eating these healthy **Wildatarian** grains may contribute to stabilizing blood sugar and lowering cholesterol—so, why not go wild with your ancient grains today?

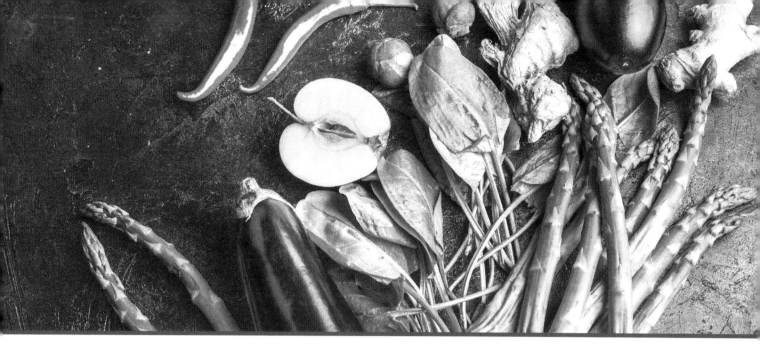

CHAPTER 7

NATURE'S WILDATARIAN GARDEN

The bounty of vegetables, herbs, and fruits from nature's garden contains deep, beautiful pigments that supply a variety of phytochemicals, antioxidants, fiber, vitamins, and minerals. The **Wildatarian** diet offers many of these, including brassica vegetables, sweet roots, herbs, avocados, and mangoes.

HEALTH BENEFITS OF THE BRASSICA VEGETABLES

Vegetables from the brassica family include arugula, bok choy, broccoli, cabbage, cauliflower, collards, kale, radishes, turnip greens, and watercress. Brassica vegetables come from the biological genus of the mustard family, and they contain sulfur. They provide a bold taste and play a role as liver detoxifiers, cancer fighters, and digestive-integrity supporters. They contain phytonutrients, specifically indole-3-carbinol (I3C), which not only help to keep our livers clear but also aid in dismantling and eliminating cancer-producing substances. Studies show that consuming these types of vegetables lowers your risk of developing lung, prostate, colon, breast, and ovarian cancers.

Hormone-driven cancers are now the fastest growing in the United States, and how we produce, store, and metabolize estrogen affects our risk. I3C helps with estrogen metabolism by promoting the conversion of the active estrogen forms and their byproducts to much safer compounds. I3C may also help block cancer-enhancing receptor sites. In a study conducted by the Department of Pathology at the Karmanos Cancer Institute in the Wayne State University School of Medicine, researchers stated, "Here we report for the first time that I3C inhibits the growth of PC-3 prostate cancer cells."

Brassica vegetables aren't just cancer fighters. Cabbage contains the amino acid L-Glutamine, which is one of the fuel sources for maintenance and repair of the cells of the stomach and small intestine. Cabbage juice is known for helping to manage ulcers. Along with removing gluten, drinking cabbage juice also played a role in restoring the gastrointestinal health of one of my clients who suffered from gastric conditions for more than twenty years. She affectionately referred to her cabbage juice as "skunk juice," as it derives its strong odor from the high sulfur content.

This vegetable family infuses its nutrients into the recipes for *Green Garden Soup* and *Chinese Wild Shrimp and Cabbage*. These recipes were created in part to provide multiple ways to use vegetables that may be wilting in your refrigerator so they don't go to waste.

Although brassicas are powerfully healing, they can be less so for individuals who have sulfur sensitivity, and I recommend avoiding these vegetables during the **Rebalance** phase of the **HealAndSeal** Program if you are a **WS–** or **WFS–TYPE**. Along the same lines, I also recommend that sulfur-sensitive individuals speak to their healthcare practitioners about supplements with sulfuric compounds such as diindolylmethane and garlic. Many try to help respiratory infections and blood sugar imbalance with these common, over-the-counter supplements without considering the possible negative implications. Our clients with sulfur sensitivity have experienced rebalancing of their symptoms by temporarily eliminating sulfur-rich foods and adding nutrients designed to improve the metabolism of sulfur.

Some of these specific nutrients include molybdenum found in chickpeas, and vitamin B6 found in grains. I personally have a sulfur sensitivity, so I need to be mindful of not overdoing sulfur-rich foods, but I can enjoy them if I am careful. When I first became a **Wildatarian**, I eliminated sulfur-containing foods altogether. Now I can consume them in moderation without a problem, because I strictly adhere to my **Wildatarian** principals. After eliminating sulfuric foods for a period, I suggest you start by reintroducing the kinder variety of sulfur veggies such as well-cooked cauliflower and broccoli. Roasted or cooked is better, but please limit raw consumption, and do not incorporate them into your juices or smoothies.

OXALATES

I touched on oxalates in Chapter 5, but because certain "healthy" vegetables may be anything but healthy for you if you have an oxalate metabolism issue, I want to mention this again.

I advise some of my clients to avoid the vegetables I consider to be higher in oxalates, which include beets, spinach, swiss chard, okra, and parsley. Abstain from them for a period of six weeks. If you feel digestive changes or experience other symptoms upon reintroduction, then stop their intake again.

SWEET ROOTS

Sweet potatoes help to satisfy my sweet tooth, and even though they are sweet tasting, they help to stabilize blood-sugar levels because of their high-fiber content. This brilliantly colored root vegetable has replaced the white potato in our home. *Sweet Potato "Fries"* included in the recipe for *Herbed Buffalo or Lamb Burgers*, are a great french-fry alternative and are actually baked, which lowers the fat content. Squash, such as butternut, summer, yellow, or zucchini, also can serve as a nice white potato substitute for roasting, in soups, or for making purées. Although sweet potato is considered a moderate oxalate-rich food, I have observed that most of my clients with an oxalate sensitivity can still consume this nutrient-rich vegetable because of its other beneficial properties, including its sugar-balancing benefits and high vitamin A content.

HERBS FOR FRESH AND NUTRITIOUS MEALS

Using herbs is an easy way to create gourmet-tasting yet simple meals. Herbs add tremendous flavor to food, and I consider them to be essential to fresh and nutritious cooking. You'll find you don't need complicated or exotic ingredients when using fresh herbs.

I cook seasonally with herbs. During the summer, I pick them from the garden for use the same day. Cilantro, parsley, basil, and rosemary are easy to grow almost anywhere, even in small spaces.

Oregano, popular in Spanish, Cuban, and Italian cuisine, is an herb I use regularly for flavoring my **Wildatarian** proteins, soups, and bean dishes.

Another big summertime herb is basil, and I incorporate it into dishes in numerous ways. Try it in *Thai Basil, Coconut, and Curry Squash Soup,* or even use it as a dessert ingredient in *Plum Boats with Basil and Goat Cheese.* Thursdays are frittata nights at our house. The flavor from fresh basil and plum tomatoes in *Tomato, Basil, and Goat Cheese Frittata* greatly enhances the eggs. I purchase fresh basil when my garden can no longer provide it.

I use herbs for more than simply flavoring dishes. One of my clients remarked that she never knew that eating an herb (cilantro) as a salad green could be so refreshing!

BENEFITS OF AVOCADO

Avocados are often not given their rightful place on the plate because of their fat content and calories. Of course, if we overindulge in any food and don't burn those calories, weight gain can result. And yes, avocados are high in fat. But the type of fat is important, and avocados are rich in the monounsaturated fat that is so good for us. Monounsaturated beneficial fats and oils are a slow-burning fuel, leaving us feeling fuller longer. Avocados also are considered an anti-estrogenic food. By helping to block estrogen absorption, they support in balancing high estrogen levels that disrupt hormones and promote weight gain.

Regular consumption of avocados is heart healthy. They help manage cholesterol levels and contain higher potassium levels than bananas. I incorporate avocados into my meal planning and preparation every week. Try them in my *Avocado, Papaya, and Cilantro Salad,* and, of course, in guacamole. You also can use avocado as a spread in sandwiches in lieu of mayonnaise. My children used to brown bag their school lunches daily and often chose avocado and spinach wraps (recipe not provided, but easy to assemble using *Herb-Rubbed Roasted Duck* or *Avocado, Tomato, and Hummus Wrap).* You can serve avocados as a side with dinner, or even for breakfast with eggs.

MIGHTY MANGO

I feature mangoes in *Mango and Black Bean Salad*. I have had a long relationship with this fruit, probably because I had mango trees in my backyard in Cuba and later in Florida. Mangoes are one of the most consumed fruits across the globe, and they come in more than fifty varieties. Studies at the University of Florida demonstrated that the compounds in mangoes exhibit anti-cancer effects. Mangoes are great blood-builders due to their high iron content, and heart healthy due to high concentrations of potassium and magnesium, making them highly alkalizing. They are also very thyroid protective as they are rich in iodine. We consider papaya to be a lower sugar fruit than mango, so substitute papaya for mango in most recipes if you want to lower the natural sugar content of your meal.

Deeply pigmented colors, and nutrients from nature's garden should be a daily staple in your **Wildatarian** fare.

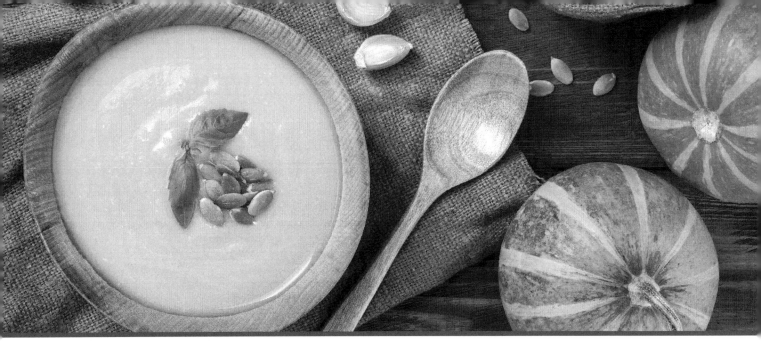

CHAPTER 8

SOUL-SATISFYING WILDATARIAN SOUPS AND BROTHS

Soups warm and nourish our bodies and souls. Few dishes can compare as a healthful comfort food. This universal one-dish meal can be served rustic or sophisticated and elegant to suit your needs. Also budget-friendly, soups can be made with ingredients already stocked in your kitchens. You even can make use of bones from the wild game in my recipes, which would otherwise be discarded. My **Wildatarian** approach embraces using the whole animal, creating abundance rather than waste.

Create delicious varieties of soup by starting with a pot of water—what is simpler and yet inspirational? You can't go wrong with making soup. If the flavor doesn't quite fit your taste buds, then just add ingredients or liquid until it does.

PEASANT-STYLE SOUPS

My soups start with straightforward ingredients: water, bones, onion, and salt. I prefer to use the bones of buffalo/bison, Cornish game hens, lamb or pheasant, but any wild bones will do. If I am making a vegetable stock, then I start with onions, salt, and pepper. From there, I add whatever vegetables, beans, grains, and herbs (fresh or dried) I have on hand. If I have collards in the refrigerator, then they eventually end up as an ingredient in soup. If you have a sulfur sensitivity, use Swiss chard instead. [7]

When soup simmers, it beautifully marries all the added flavors. Moreover, soup is an easy way to get animal protein, greens, beans, and grains from one bowl of piping-hot goodness. This meal also provides a lower-fat method of cooking, for those whose **Wildatarian** type limits fats. Making soups allows you to use vegetables that are no longer crisp enough for salads, but are not yet spoiled. Just drop cilantro, parsley, and broccoli into some hot water and you have the makings of my *Green Garden Soup*, which is especially bountiful in antioxidants, chlorophyll, and anti-cancer agents. Again, use your **Wildatarian** type to determine what to include in your soup.

SILKY SOUPS

For more sophisticated soups, I use an immersion blender to purée the cooked ingredients. A regular blender or food processor will work just as well. Puréeing gives soup a gourmet texture. For cream-based soups, I do not use cow's milk or cream. I opt instead for coconut, goat, or sheep milk, making the soup more easily digestible for those with a cow-dairy sensitivity. *Thai Basil, Coconut, and Curry Squash Soup* is a great example of a silky soup. The flavors that these milk replacements lend to soups are outstanding. Adding a dollop of goat cheese increases their creaminess.

Many of my convertible dishes start or end with soup. Sometimes, it's bean soup or maybe just a simple broth. When creating a convertible dish, just double the amount of meat or beans you use and save half to be incorporated into a future recipe (see *Wild Boar Carnitas, Cuban Ropa*

---

7   Collards are a signature ingredient in Galician soups as they are for mine. Peasant soups connect me to my Spanish ancestral roots—my great-grandfather was a Galician cook. The cold and wet climate of Galicia, located in northwest Spain, calls for soups.

Vieja, Cuban Black Beans, and bean-based appetizers). Otherwise, try starting with another dish such as the *Herb-Rubbed Roasted Duck*, and end up with soup.

I usually make soup on Sundays, a day that for me tends to be a little lazier and gives me the luxury of time to make this type of meal. I double the recipe so I have enough for additional meals during the week. Sometimes during the winter, I eat soup for breakfast! Alternatively, the soup can be spooned into individual serving containers and frozen for easy, healthful, take-to-work meals.

Soup is also my go-to meal when I am really short on time, because I typically keep a large container of it in the freezer—though it is important to date any food you prepare and freeze. There is such a sense of comfort knowing that my trusty soup is there and waiting to be thawed. I add a salad and some healthy bread, and dinner is served. There's no need to make the "drive of shame" (a phrase coined by one of my clients) to a fast-food establishment. These options allow for fast, convenient, and healthful foods right in your kitchen.

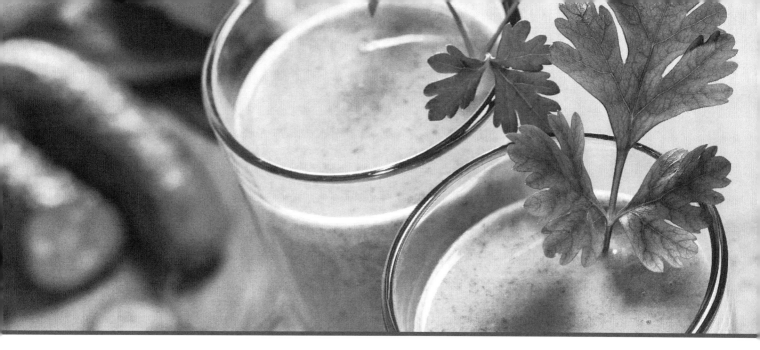

CHAPTER 9

WILDATARIAN-STYLE JUICING AND BEVERAGES

When most Americans drink a beverage these days, it more than likely contains high fructose corn syrup (HFCS), artificial sweeteners such as Splenda and Sweet'N Low (many of which have been linked to cancer and diabetes), artificial colors, artificial flavors, preservatives, and very little else.

Fruit drinks and even most fruit juices list HFCS as their first ingredient. These types of beverages do nothing to support health and, in fact, may contribute to disease. They are among the main culprits in increasing acidity, inflammation, and blood sugar levels, all of which may lead to diabetes, obesity, and other chronic conditions. Even "healthful" smoothies may be full of sugar and be anything but healthy. Let me show you how to change what you drink from a disease promoter to a disease fighter.

I offer a selection of homemade juices, smoothies, tea blends, and naturally flavored waters that may help boost energy, alkalize and oxygenate the body, stabilize blood sugar levels, and soothe

the nervous system. The Standard American Diet is inflammatory in nature, and promotes disease. My libations offer supportive nutrients, antioxidants, phytonutrients, and oxygen-rich chlorophyll.

WILDATARIAN-STYLE JUICING

I highlight green juices, because of the extraordinary health benefits they contain. Why green? One of my mantras is to "Go Green and Get Clean." Green because deep green vegetables are rich in chlorophyll—the compound that gives plants this beautiful color.

AMAZING CHLOROPHYLL

Chlorophyll, rich in magnesium and iron, can act as a cleanser, an internal healing agent, a rejuvenator, a builder of red blood cells, and a liver detoxifier. Chlorophyll is the "blood" of plants and very closely resembles human blood. Dr. Richard Willstätter, a German chemist who was awarded the 1915 Nobel Prize for chemistry, found that the chlorophyll molecule is quite similar to hemoglobin, the oxygen carrier in our blood. Magnesium promotes a state of alkalinity, and iron further enriches the blood, because it works with protein to make hemoglobin in red blood cells.

The chlorophyll we ingest through green vegetables helps to oxygenate our bodies and promote healthy cellular function. These green "giants" are rich in folate, vitamin C, and potassium. They also contain a host of phytochemicals such as lutein and beta-carotene. Disease is less likely to live in an oxygen-rich, alkaline environment. The human body and all its tissues are most optimal at around 7.2 pH. Otherwise, a condition wherein the body becomes overly acidic ensues. Many studies have shown that acute acidosis can cause bacteria, yeast, and fungus to take over and spark degenerative diseases including, diabetes, cancer, arteriosclerosis, and chronic fatigue.

BENEFITS OF JUICING

Juicing breaks down the plant's cell walls, making it easier for someone with impaired digestive function to receive the vegetable's health benefits. This delivery system gives the digestive tract a respite from the work of breaking down high-fiber foods to extract their nutrients. As a result, highly concentrated nutrients go directly into the system—like a nutrition IV.

Juicing has all of the benefits of eating whole vegetables except that it lacks fiber. If you also want fiber, then make a smoothie instead or use the pulp from your juice extraction in soups, breads, and smoothies. Nothing should be thrown away. That's the **Wildatarian** way.

I have chosen simple green juices to get you started, and these are shared in my recipe section. My *Cilantro and Cucumber Juice (BYOJ)*, which I drink daily, is the easiest on your gut, so I suggest that it be your entry into the world of juicing. These ingredients are both sulfur- and oxalate-free.

Start with one bunch of cilantro rinsed and two peeled cucumbers. Juice and enjoy. As you build your own juice (BYOJ) combinations, be mindful—you want your tummy to feel good after drinking them. You should dilute your juice by a two-to-one ratio with water. If you feel queasy or nauseous as you start making different combinations, then back down and drink less of the juice, add more water, or change your combination of vegetables. The reason you may feel a little queasy is because these deep green juices are potent liver detoxifiers. Little digestion is needed as the juices go directly to work. This can be somewhat taxing if your liver dumps toxins into a system that is not ready to handle them. If this is the case for you, flu-like symptoms may follow, so it is best to start slowly.

I usually recommend two ounces of juice to four ounces of water. You still will get the health benefits from the plant nutrients, but will do so in a gentler way. Once your body adjusts, you can drink the undiluted juice. You don't need a lot of juice—four ounces daily is a good goal to achieve.

As you add the deeper-colored and more bitter greens to your juicing blends, consider adding lemon juice or apple cider vinegar. Just a quarter teaspoon is enough to get you started. Then you can decide how much your palate likes. (I recommend no more than one tablespoon, because these ingredients can affect your tooth enamel.) My clients find that the juice makes their bodies feel so good that they don't mind the taste of even the most bitter of greens; they associate the juice with how great it makes them feel.

Once you get the hang of juicing, you'll be amazed by how many different, delicious, and satisfying combinations you can create. In general, favor vegetables over fruits when juicing to minimize blood-sugar implications. With fruit, when you eliminate the fiber, you have a concentrated form of sugar (I save my fruits for smoothies). Remember, these juices go directly to work in your system.

Important note: If you have sulfur sensitivities, then it is extremely important that you **do not juice** with sulfur-containing greens and foods. These include:

- arugula
- bok choy
- broccolini
- broccoli
- Brussels sprouts
- cabbage
- cauliflower
- celery
- collard greens
- dandelion root
- garlic
- kale
- leeks
- onion
- radish/daikon
- shallots
- watercress

WILDATARIAN SMOOTHIES

Inviting Smoothies are great fruit combinations that can also be frozen and made into sorbet-like treats—a great alternative to fatty and cow-milk-based ice cream. The ingredients in these smoothies provide an array of vitamins, antioxidants, and protein.

With juices and smoothies, you can greatly increase your vegetable and fruit intake. I strongly encourage you to choose organic produce, and especially avoid the items on the Environmental Working Group's Dirty Dozen list, which you will find at ewg.org/foodnews/dirty_dozen_list.php.

The average American consumes more than five pounds of pesticides and herbicides in food each year. Toxic chemicals should not be part of the cocktail you create. By using organic produce, you will minimize these toxins.

Smoothies are a great afternoon treat for kids. A few starter recipes have been provided, but you can create your own. Your smoothie universe is as large as the selection of fruits available at your farmers market or natural grocer. Include mild-tasting greens to inject additional phytonutrients without having to fight the kids to eat them.

WILDATARIAN TEA BLENDS

Tea blends are great coolers. Some tea blends feature mint—an herb with many beneficial properties. It has been shown to relieve symptoms of irritable bowel syndrome, including indigestion and colonic muscle spasms. Chamomile, another tea staple, may be beneficial in soothing the stomach and relaxing the nervous system, and has been shown to contain anti-inflammatory properties[8].

Green tea is a good alternative to other caffeinated beverages because it contains approximately thirty milligrams of caffeine per serving, a little less than half that of coffee. One cup of green tea may have a greater antioxidant effect than a serving of broccoli, spinach, carrots, or strawberries. This high-antioxidant content may help protect our bodies from damage caused by free radicals—a byproduct of cellular function that can create oxidative stress and change the structure of cell membranes, making them susceptible to damage[9].

Sip and enjoy. Another **Wildatarian** way to support better health.

---

8   If you are allergic to ragweed, then do not over consume chamomile, as it is a botanical cousin and may increase your allergy symptoms during ragweed season. Stay away from mint if you have ulcers or GERD, because it may increase symptoms related to them.

9   Drinking green tea is contraindicated for multiple myeloma patients who are taking bortezomib.

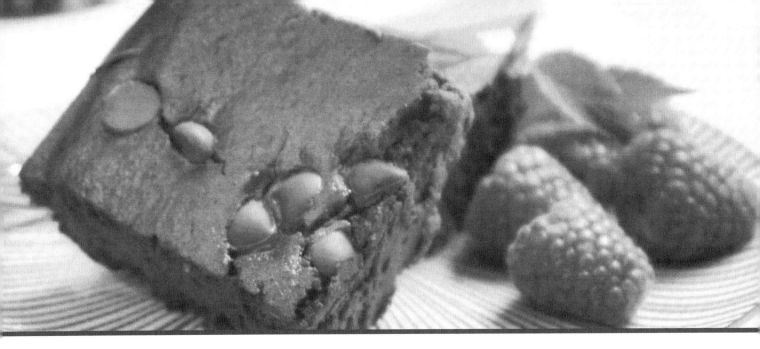

CHAPTER 10

GOING WILD WITH DESSERTS AND SAVORY TREATS

Desserts and savory treats do not have to be excluded when following the **Wildatarian** approach and lifestyle. Eliminating sweets is a form of deprivation that cannot be sustained, and it often backfires in the long run. Ultimately, shifting the way we think about what defines a dessert or sweet treat is what will allow us to make healthful choices.

Unless you have a health condition that prohibits the consumption of simple sugars in any form, it is perfectly acceptable for you to enjoy something sweet every now and then. In fact, consuming natural sugars at the end of the meal can signal the brain to turn off its appetite response. The problem is that commercially made sweet breads, muffins, pies, cookies, cakes, and puddings typically have little to offer in the way of nutrition. They feature refined flours and high fructose corn syrup as prominent ingredients, followed by artificial flavors, food dyes, preservatives such as sulfites and sulfates, and other unhealthy constituents.

Originally, desserts were intended to be small and delicate morsels reserved for the end of a special meal. Today, a supersized, gooey, and cake-like muffin—packed with more sugar and fat than desserts of the past—is considered not just for dessert but also as an acceptable breakfast option. **Wildatarian** breakfasts include yummy options such as bars, pancakes, and muffins, but without all the sugar and unacceptable ingredients.

READY FOR DESSERT?

Meals should end when you are about 80 percent satiated, as it takes approximately twenty minutes for the nerve endings in the stomach to signal the brain that the stomach is full. Not becoming overfull leaves the physical space your stomach needs to properly mix the ingested food with acid and enzymes, and facilitates optimal digestion. If you eat too quickly or if you continue eating to the point of feeling full, you have overeaten. Eating slowly and only until you are just satiated is a healthy habit to practice for fostering a healthy gut biome—and it will leave room for a correctly portioned, end-of-meal treat.

DESSERT INGREDIENTS AND COMPONENTS

When I read food labels, I subscribe to a general rule: if the ingredients cannot be pronounced, they should not go into my body. This is a "can't read it, won't eat it" approach: the body also can't "read" such ingredients to properly digest and assimilate them. Most listed ingredients ending with -ite or -ate or difficult-to-pronounce food additives are antithetical to the **Wildatarian** approach. In addition, foods that are high in sugar feed systemic yeast and bacteria, which causes and/or exacerbates gut impairment. As a **Wildatarian**, you should learn to read food labels to avoid these toxins.

The **Wildatarian** desserts and savory recipes included in this book support my philosophy around sweets. Protein, fats, and carbohydrates are absorbed at different rates in the digestive tract. Research shows that if you are going to take in a carbohydrate-dense food, then you should pair it with a protein or fat.

DESSERT PAIRINGS

My favorite dessert pairings with naturally sweetened treats include raw nuts, seeds, goat and sheep milk cheeses, dark chocolate, and coconut and almond milks. If you have an oxalate issue, then you can substitute either hemp, sheep, or brown rice milk for the coconut and almond milks. But how do you turn these ingredients into a dessert? My recipes will show you easy ways to create a dessert that will leave you feeling great while satisfying your sweet tooth.

When having something sweet, like chocolate, I almost always add nuts or seeds. I alternate bites of chocolate with bites of almonds, walnuts, hazelnuts, or sunflower seeds. This smooths out chocolate's bittersweet flavor while offering the protein and fat my body needs to slow the absorption of the chocolate's sugar.

Additionally, combining fruit, nuts, seeds, and honey is a simple and sweet way to end any meal. You will navigate which of these suit you best based on your **Wildatarian** type. I often pair papaya, tangerine, or mango slices with chopped almonds, walnuts, or pumpkin seeds, and then top it with goat cheese and honey to add texture and sweetness. Just about any nut and fruit combination works well. I encourage you to experiment to find what best fits your palate preference. *Plum Boats with Basil and Goat Cheese* deliver a combination of sweet and savory flavors.

To enjoy healthful versions of more traditional desserts, including pie, cake, brownies, or rice and bread puddings, I use the **Wildatarian** grains of brown rice, oats, quinoa, and buckwheat. *Fruit and Nut Bread Pudding* combines many of my favorite flavors with its nuts, coconut, and dried fruit. *Wild Blueberry, Quinoa, and Oat Bars* and *Banana, Buckwheat, and Chocolate Chip Muffins* are reminiscent of cake and ice cream, but they do not have all the fatty and heavy ingredients.

Reap the benefits of consuming nature's sweet nectar from nuts, seeds, fruits, and honey, and healthy whole-grain treats instead of heavy and rich desserts that are nutrient-poor and calorie-rich (which will deregulate your blood sugar and potentially affect your epigenetics). These desserts will leave you satisfied but not overly full—and your new **Wildatarian** body will thank you.

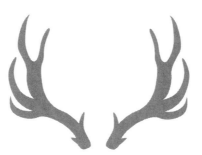

ACKNOWLEDGMENTS

I would like to thank everyone who took part in the creation and publishing of this book, especially Margo Kirzhner and Sarah Devido, who researched and contributed to the body and work of this book, Lindsay Benson Garrett for her design, photography, and branding skills, and Candace Johnson for her editing skills.

And thanks to all who touched this work to bring it to you so that it may have a positive impact in your life, especially William Cochrane, Madeleine Cochrane, Lauren Rice, and Joelle Shreves.

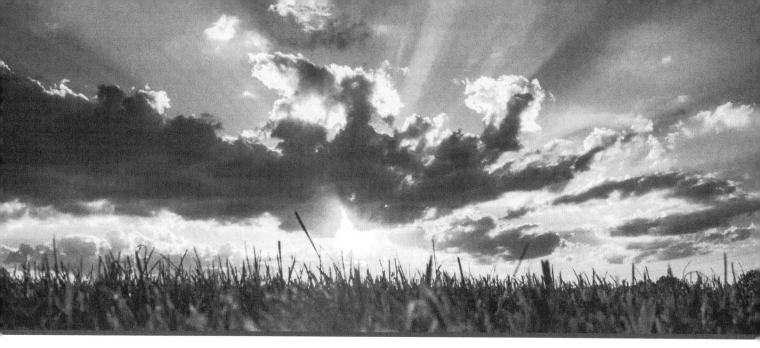

WILDATARIAN STORIES OF TRANSFORMATION

My philosophy is that if I ask the right questions, the correct answers will follow. I have developed a methodology of bio-individualized plans for my clients that blends the latest in cutting-edge science, biomechanics, observation, listening, and nutrition, because everyone is different. What may work for you may not work for your neighbor, spouse, or friends. The **Wildatarian** diet and **HealAndSeal** Program aim to guide you to your individual needs.

My clients faced many health challenges, including chronic conditions involving thyroid imbalance, digestive problems, food allergies and intolerance, endocrine disfunction (difficulty conceiving and weight gain), mood changes, anxiety, and other challenges. The following are testimonials from just a few of these transformative stories.

A WILDATARIAN LIFESTYLE IN CONJUNCTION WITH CHEMOTHERAPY FOR AMYLOIDOSIS: FORTY-FOUR-YEAR-OLD CANCER PATIENT GLENN ENJOYS REMISSION

At the risk of sounding overly dramatic, Teri taught us that food can be the difference between life and death. Four-and-a-half years ago, my husband was diagnosed with a rare form of blood cancer called amyloidosis. The disease deposits sticky protein cells in the major organs of the body. In my husband's case, it was primarily his heart. The day before he was to start chemo, he had a stroke and was in the hospital for a month. During that time, I begged for information about how to support my husband through nutrition, but the doctors could only encourage me to do so. They had no concrete guidance. During my husband's convalescence at home, friends brought us meals, including one from Teri's cookbook. I booked an appointment with Teri and my husband's road to recovery began.

Teri taught us that it is important to not only eat healthy food, but to be able to distinguish which food is helpful and which is not. Something got my husband to the point of desperate ill health, and in that state, even some 'healthy foods' could be harmful. Teri was able to identify what he needed to cut out and what he needed to eat more of. By all accounts, my husband should not be alive today. He's been in remission for two-and-a-half years; he's working and he's riding his bike daily. We continue to eat healthy, and though the doctors tell us the cancer will return again, we believe that through healthy eating, he will continue to defy the odds.

THE WILDATARIAN APPROACH TO LYME DISEASE FOR FORTY-YEAR-OLD ERIKA

Before I visited Teri Cochrane, I doubted that any nutritionist could help me. I suffered terribly from Lyme and associated diseases for eight years, and saw many practitioners of both conventional and alternative therapies, even traveling all over the United States and internationally to see the top practitioners. After many years, they were able to stop the progress of the disease, but could not help me get my health back.

So, when someone recommended that I see Teri, I was not optimistic. But Teri is different from the typical practitioner who might have treated you in the past. At my first visit, Teri went back to the basics in terms of nutrition. I needed to be a low fat, low sulfur Wildatarian.

I am convinced that Teri's nutritional protocol was the missing link. The plan she recommended was very effective in supporting my health.

TWENTY-SEVEN-YEAR-OLD MUSIC TEACHER WITH UNDIFFERENTIATED CONNECTIVE TISSUE DISORDER FINDS HEALTH AGAIN USING A WILDATARIAN APPROACH

I saw Teri at the end of May 2016. I had been on steroids and arthritis medicine consistently for pain management since September of 2015, and on and off since the fall of 2009. I had been dealing with a mysterious flare-up that came and went. The flare-up started in my hands with severe and debilitating pain and swelling, but would eventually spread to other major joints and even into the muscles. By January 2016, I was bedridden. Picking up something as small and lightweight as a toothbrush became a daily challenge. I had consulted with multiple rheumatologists, chiropractors, acupuncturists, internal medicine doctors ... just about everyone. I felt hopeless and was dealing with symptoms of anxiety and depression.

Teri put me on a Wildatarian plan and nutritional protocol to help cleanse my body of toxins that had built up over the years. She instilled a new hope in me the first day that I visited her office. In just about eight weeks of being on the regimen, I started to feel improvement. It felt like a miracle! Eight years of pain and unknown circumstances to eight weeks, and I felt improvement!

I have had friends and family tell me that I look better and they can tell I have that 'spring in my step' back! Teri takes her time to look at the whole person and consider all of you.

CLIENT WITH CHRONIC PAIN FINDS RELIEF FOLLOWING WILDATARIAN PLAN

Spine surgery gone wrong, a physical assault in a foreign country, and a couple of other traumatic life events left me with sciatica, anxiety, and chronic pain, which began in February 2012 and remained with me for four solid years. When I woke up each morning, my first thought was always, how bad will it hurt today? Pain was always on my mind. It sapped my energy and took away my ability to think clearly. It defined me. I was no longer a forty-something-year-old wife, mother, daughter, and friend, but a person in severe pain who could sometimes barely walk, sit down, or find any comfortable position. The only remedy involved a sleeping pill and going to bed. I wondered how many more years I would live, and whether chronic pain could actually kill a person. My feet hurt. My back ached. My mouth and swollen tongue felt like they were on fire.

I did everything I could think of to erase the pain. I saw more doctors—spine surgeons, neurosurgeons, mental health professionals, and pain specialists. I had X-rays, MRIs, EMGs, blood tests, and many, many different types of injections. I tried prolotherapy (considered experimental and not covered by insurance) and ordered various remedies, such as back braces, menthol creams, and e-stim devices. I took anti-inflammatories, muscle spasm medication, and every type of painkiller I could find (or that doctors would allow), but nothing worked, and no two doctors could agree on why I was in so much pain. Outwardly, I tried to act and appear normal, if only for the sake of my family, friends, and co-workers.

I will never forget the day one of my doctors scoffed, 'There's nothing wrong with you. You look too good to be in pain,' as he shooed me out of his office. The following week, I found out I had a torn hip labrum, yet another ailment to add to my list.

Thousands of dollars, hundreds of hours, and four years later, I met Teri, and this changed my life.

I finally had days where I woke up in the morning thinking about things other than pain. In fact, some days I even forgot about the pain. Today, I rarely even think about pain, because for the most part, it is gone! My heels don't hurt any longer, and I can wear normal shoes again. I can sit for hours at a time without getting a backache. My mouth looks and feels good. My thoughts are no longer cloudy, and I am not as forgetful, jumpy, or moody. I have more energy and feel great. One of my best friends recently told me that I looked different, but couldn't quite figure out why. She said my skin and face looked good, and she even asked me who I was seeing for cosmetic surgery. I laughed and told her the truth—the difference was attributable to Teri and her bio-individual Wildatarian plan, not a plastic surgeon!

OLYMPIC HOPEFUL RESOLVES COMPLETE BODY HAIR LOSS AND BREAKS HER PERSONAL RECORDS

Madelyn came to my practice as a twelve-year-old girl, a high-level competitive long-distance swimmer who was experiencing alopecia totalis, an autoimmune condition with varying degrees of hair loss. For Madelyn, this meant total body hair loss, including her beautiful head of hair. Her symptoms began in September 2012, and within five months, she had complete hair loss. It started to come back but fell out again in May of 2013. She then started pharmaceutical treatment.

Her doctors' approach was to give Madelyn steroid shots in her head and have her take oral steroids as well as apply a topical steroidal cream. The steroid cream irritated her skin. The steroid shots were terribly painful.

It was at this time she decided to seek natural approaches to health and came to my office at the recommendation of her dermatologist. During the initial consultation and by looking at Madelyn's body as a whole, I was able to come up with a plan to support this promising athlete. I recommended a wholesome food plan and supplements[10] to balance her system and support her gut integrity. After nine months, her hair grew back and she started breaking records for her age group.

10 Madelyn's supplements were approved through the Olympic Committee so as not to be considered illegally enhancing. In addition, she was not able to provide testimony due to the NCAA rules governing endorsements.

Eighteen months later, Madelyn experienced a setback, and she started to lose her hair again. We then had Madelyn follow her **Wildatarian** food plan. Her hair grew back over a period of months. She is now ranked in the top 100 in the world (eighteen and under) as a distance swimmer.

WILDATARIAN FOOD PLAN HELPS BREASTFEEDING MOTHER PROVIDE HEALING NUTRIENTS TO NEWBORN SON

It is a great privilege to share my healing story. Teri has seen me, my husband, and my children over the last five years. Because of our previous experiences with Teri and her success in working with my family, when I became pregnant with my fourth child, I made an appointment with her at twenty-four weeks to determine what foods and diet would be best for my developing baby. She determined that I would need to stick to a gluten-free meat and veggies diet, low in sugar and sulfur. I happily changed my diet that evening.

My baby was born healthy and happy, but at four months old became constipated, could barely pass a bowel movement, and started to lose weight. Since I still was exclusively breastfeeding him, this was very alarming. I knew something in my diet was affecting his ability to digest my milk properly and I immediately set up an appointment with Teri. At that visit, she determined quickly that his little body was unable to tolerate most animal proteins. Teri placed me (because he was only consuming my breast milk) on the Wildatarian protocol and I continued to be gluten and sulfur free. Within three days of changing my diet, he was back to passing his bowel movements with ease on a regular schedule.

I continued to exclusively breastfeed and eat this Wildatarian diet and began introducing solid foods to William at ten months. I am proud to say he is now an energetic and inquisitive fifteen-month-old child.

These clients found their individual truth. Our practice gives people hope that a holistic and individualized nutritional and lifestyle approach can help restore balance and well-being.

DISCLAIMER

The client stories featured in this section are provided for informational and educational purposes only. The statements made, and the results described herein, relate only to limited, individualized experiences of these selected clients. This information is not intended to represent or suggest that following the **Wildatarian** diet or the **HealAndSeal** Program will produce a similar result for you, or that either program will benefit you in any way. Every individual is unique, and there is no single dietary or nutritional protocol that works for everyone. This information is not intended as medical advice, and is not intended to represent or imply that the **Wildatarian** food plan or any nutritional protocol described herein is recommended for use in the diagnosis, cure, mitigation, treatment or prevention of any disease. We primarily use food and body observation in our practice to guide people in their search for optimal health and wellness. In doing so, we abide by the philosophy of "Let food be thy medicine."

GLOSSARY

90/10

A food plan in which the 90 stands for "90 percent sensible food choices" and the 10 for "10 percent fringe food choices;" this food plan allows for some flexibility and indulgence

Acid

A substance that has a pH lower than 7; the lower a substance's pH, the greater the acidity level

Adrenal fatigue

A collection of symptoms—including body aches, general fatigue, nervousness, trouble sleeping, digestive problems, and lightheadedness—that usually indicate the adrenals are not functioning properly or producing hormones efficiently

Adrenal glands

Endocrine glands found above the kidneys that produce a variety of hormones, including adrenaline and steroids, such as aldosterone and cortisol; these can be inordinately affected by the ever-present chronic stress in our modern lifestyle

Aflatoxins

A group of toxins produced by fungi that is typically found on certain crops like corn, peanuts, cottonseed, and tree nuts. These have been found to be cancer promoting and increase likelihood of allergic responses in predisposed individuals

Alkaline food

A food that balances the pH level of bodily fluids like blood and urine; many fruits, vegetables, as well as some nuts, seeds, and legumes, are alkaline-promoting foods

Alkalization

The process of making something more basic (maintaining a pH greater than 7)

Allergen
A type of antigen that produces an abnormal immune response, in which the immune system fights off a perceived threat

Alzheimer's disease
A progressive disease that destroys memory and other important mental functions

Amino acid
The basic building block of protein in the body, which is capable of forming tissues, organs, muscles, skin, and hair; amino acids are also sources of energy in the body, along with fats and carbohydrates

Ammonia
A compound formed in the body when protein is broken down in the gut, which is then converted to urea by the liver and excreted as urine; when the liver is unable to convert ammonia to urea for excretion, the ammonia level in the blood rises

Amyloidosis
A rare disease that occurs when misfolded proteins called amyloids build up in organs; severe amyloidosis can lead to life-threatening organ failure

Amyloid
Aggregate of proteins that become folded into a functional shape, which allows many copies of this new mis-formed protein to stick together and form fibrils; amyloids may contribute to various diseases as previously healthy proteins lose their normal physiological functions and form fibrous deposits in plaques around cells; these plaques disrupt the healthy function of tissues and organs; our bodies have some ability to break down amyloids, but when maintenance mechanisms in the body can no longer manage their breakdown, a disease state may ensue

Ancient grain
A group of grains not considered to be denatured

Antibiotic

A class of antimicrobial drugs that either kills or prevents the growth of bacteria and is, therefore used to treat bacterial infections in the body; antibiotics are widely used in animal agriculture; antibiotics may disrupt a healthy gut biome

Antibody

A large protein made by the body's immune system to neutralize different pathogens like bacteria and viruses

Antioxidant

A substance that inhibits oxidation (stress/rust/damage) in the body; substances like vitamins C and E, and minerals like selenium and zinc can act like antioxidants in the body; some foods rich in antioxidants are considered superfoods

APOE gene

A gene family that provides instructions for making a protein that helps regulate cholesterol and certain fats in the body; some variants in this gene family have been linked with Alzheimer's disease

Assimilation

The absorption and digestion of food or nutrients by the body

Asthma

A respiratory condition that causes spasms of the bronchi in the lungs and difficulty breathing

Attention deficit hyperactivity disorder (ADHD)

A chronic condition that is characterized by attention difficulty, hyperactivity, and impulsiveness

Autoimmune disorder

A class of disorders where the body's immune system mistakenly attacks and destroys healthy body tissue; there are more than eighty types of autoimmune conditions; examples include multiple sclerosis, Hashimoto's thyroiditis, and lupus

Bacteria

A large group of single-celled microorganisms, some of which may cause infections and disease in animals and humans

Ballerina syndrome

A syndrome that results from the overproduction of epinephrine, which causes the tight junctions of intestinal walls to be weakened and punctured; this state creates inflammation in the body; excess epinephrine can also cause liver congestion, which makes it harder to process fats and other fat-soluble molecules, such as estrogen; term coined by Teri Cochrane

Bioavailability

The proportion of a drug, supplement, or other substance that enters the circulation when introduced into the body and is able to have an active effect

Biochemistry

A branch of chemistry that focuses on the chemical processes that occur within the body

Biofilm

A gel-like coating that protects organisms from external dangers; pathogenic bacteria can form biofilm, which protects them against antibiotic or antimicrobial therapy

Bio-individuality

A theory stating that each body is unique and, therefore, there is no one right diet that works for everyone all of the time

Biome

A large, naturally occurring community of bacteria, viruses, and fungi occupying a habitat; the body contains several biomes, with the one occurring in the digestive tract being the most well-studied

Bleached flour

A product resulting from a chemical process to make flour appear whiter

Bloating

Any abnormal gas or swelling that typically causes an increase in the size of the abdominal area

Blood-brain barrier

A membrane that separates the blood circulating throughout the body from the extracellular fluid found in the brain and central nervous system; this membrane is highly selective and semipermeable

Body interpreter

A person who detects and interprets imbalances in the body through multilevel analyses using a variety of techniques; term coined by Teri Cochrane

Bone broth

A savory liquid that results from boiling animal bones in water for a prolonged period of time; this broth is rich in collagen and other nutrient-dense substances pulled from the bones

Cupcaking yourself

Overproduction of internal sugar and fat such as epinephrine and cortisol; the body responds similarly to eating sweets and fats (like a cupcake) with an over-secretion of insulin to lower the sugar produced; term coined by Teri Cochrane

CBS

A gene family that provides instructions for the enzyme cystathionine beta-synthase, which plays an important role in homocysteine and sulfur metabolism; the CBS gene is also an important part of the chemical pathway that breaks down sulfur in the body

Calcification

The accumulation of calcium salts in a bodily tissue; calcification normally occurs during bone formation; improper calcifications have been linked to cardiovascular disease and arthritis

Candida

A yeast-like parasitic fungus that is present in the intestines of the human body but when overgrown can cause disease. It can also be present in other parts of the body as well as in vaginal yeast infections; candida overgrowth can cause a variety of health issues

Cell membrane

A selectively permeable lipid bilayer that separates the inside of the cell from the outside environment in order to protect the cell

Chemical sensitivity

When a person's body has trouble detoxifying from a certain chemical or class of chemicals, usually due to improper function of certain detoxification pathways or lack of key nutrients

Coffee/caffeine sensitivity

The presence of overdose symptoms, such as jitteriness, insomnia, and elevated heart rate, when just a small amount of coffee or caffeine is consumed; this usually indicates that the body has trouble detoxifying or metabolizing caffeine

Commensal bacteria

Refers to bacteria living in a relationship in which one organism derives food or benefits from another organism without hurting or helping it; much of the bacteria in our digestive tract and other body biomes is commensal

COMT gene

A gene family that provides the instructions for the production of an enzyme, catechol-O-methyltransferase; this enzyme helps regulate the levels of certain hormones and neurotransmitters in the body and brain

Counterseasonal eating

Eating or incorporating certain foods in the diet when they are not in season, or not currently being grown to minimize toxic burden on the body; term coined by Teri Cochrane

Crohn's disease

A chronic inflammatory bowel disease that causes inflammation in the lining of the digestive tract, leading to abdominal discomfort, fatigue, diarrhea, weight loss and potential malnutrition

Crucifers (cruciferous vegetables)

A term for vegetables in the family Brassicaceae (including cauliflower, cabbage, garden cress, bok choy, and broccoli)

Cyanocobalamin

A synthetic form of vitamin B12 that is typically included in supplements; for people with certain genetic polymorphisms, such as in the MTHFR family, ingesting this form can be harmful

Cytochrome P450

A family of genes that is an important component of the phase 1 liver detoxification pathway; the enzymes produced by these genes help break down potentially toxic compounds and other dangerous substances in the liver

Delayed sensitivity

A secondary cellular response that typically appears 48 to 72 hours after antigen/allergen exposure

Detoxification

The way in which the body purges chemicals and toxins, including those produced from within the body and those from the external environment

Detoxification pathway in the body

A bodily process designed to break down different types of harmful or unnecessary molecules that need to be transformed and excreted; these pathways can be regulated by genes, lifestyle, toxins, diet, and supplementation; a pathway implies a multistep process where one step depends on another

Diabetes

A disease in which the body's ability to produce or respond to the hormone insulin is impaired, resulting in abnormal metabolism of carbohydrates and proteins and elevated levels of glucose in the blood and urine

Digestibility

The ability of the digestive tract to break down and assimilate food

Domesticated animal agriculture

Wild animals adapted for human consumption

Dysbiosis

A microbial imbalance or maladaptation inside the body, such as an impaired balance of bacteria, viruses, and fungi in the digestive microbiome

Eczema

An inflammation or irritation of the skin that forms an itchy rash, usually appearing dry, reddish, and scaly

Edema

Swelling caused by excess fluid trapped in your body's tissues

Endocrine system

A system that includes all the glands of the body and the hormones produced by those glands

Enriched food

A food product that contains added nutrients, including those sometimes previously extracted from the food during the denaturing process; enrichment is usually mandated by government authorities or performed to make products more marketable

Epigenetics

Any process that alters gene activity without changing the DNA sequence itself; epigenetics demonstrate how our lifestyle changes the expression of our genes; known or suspected drivers behind epigenetic processes include food, heavy metals, pesticides, diesel exhaust, tobacco smoke, polycyclic aromatic hydrocarbons, hormones, radioactivity, viruses, bacteria, basic nutrients, and stress

Epinephrine

A hormone secreted by the medulla of the adrenal glands; epinephrine is also known as adrenaline; this hormone is associated with stress

Epinephrine push

A condition in which epinephrine is released into the bloodstream due to strong emotions, such as fear or anger; this causes an increase in heart rate, muscle strength, blood pressure, and sugar metabolism; term coined by Teri Cochrane

Epstein-Barr virus (EBV)

A virus commonly known to cause the infection mononucleosis (or mono)

Essential amino acid

An acid required for biological processes, which cannot be made by the body, and as a result, must come from food; the nine essential amino acids are: histidine, isoleucine, leucine, lysine, methionine, phenylalanine, threonine, tryptophan, and valine

Essential fatty acid (EFA)

A fatty acid required for biological processes, which humans and other animals must ingest, because the body requires it for good health but cannot synthesize it

Fat malabsorption syndrome

A disorder in which the small intestine cannot absorb enough fat from the diet; improper liver or gallbladder function can also contribute to this

Fat metabolism

The biochemical process by which fats are broken down, incorporated, and used by the cells of the body

Fat soluble vitamins

Vitamins A, D, E, and K, which are stored in the body for long periods of time and generally pose a risk for toxicity when consumed in excess but are necessary for many biological functions of the body

Feeding the beast

Eating food or experiencing a stress response that may contribute or exacerbate disease in the body; term coined by Teri Cochrane

Fermentation

The chemical breakdown of a substance by bacteria, yeasts, or other microorganisms

Fire-starter

A certain food or trigger that can heighten a problem in the body or cause a resurgence of a previous disease or physical issue; term coined by Teri Cochrane

Foggy head

A sensation or state that makes it difficult for a person to think clearly, usually characterized by confusion, forgetfulness, and lack of mental focus or clarity

Fungal/fungus

A fungus is any member of the group of eukaryotic organisms that includes microorganisms such as yeasts and molds, as well as mushrooms

Gene

A unit of heredity that is transferred from a parent to offspring and is held to determine some characteristic of the offspring

Gene expression

The process by which possession of a gene leads to the expression of its characteristics in the body; genes can be expressed or de-expressed by epigenetic processes

Genetic predisposition

An increased likelihood of developing a particular trait or disease based on a person's genetic makeup

Genetically modified (GM) food

Food produced from organisms that have had changes introduced into their DNA using the methods of genetic engineering

Glucose metabolism

The process of maintaining proper blood glucose levels and breaking down carbohydrates into energy for the body

Glyphosate

An herbicide and the active ingredient in the popular Roundup weed killer that is typically sprayed on crops in the United States

Goitrogen

A substance that disrupts the production of thyroid hormones by interfering with iodine uptake in the thyroid gland

Hashimoto's thyroiditis

An autoimmune disease in which the immune system turns against the body's own tissues or enzymes, specifically having to do with thyroid function

HCL (hydrochloric acid)

A strong, corrosive, and irritating acid that is normally present in a diluted form in gastric juice; this acid helps disarm pathogens in food and is key to proper breakdown of proteins in the diet; HCL levels are negatively affected by age, improper eating practices, bacteria, and protein pump inhibitor (PPI) medications such as Zantac and Prilosec

HealAndSeal™ Program

A process and program by which damaged gut lining is rebalanced and then "sealed" through a combination of bio-individualized, nutrient-dense foods and lifestyle modifications; term coined by Teri Cochrane

Helper B

Methylated B vitamins that act as co-enzymes to help neurotransmitters cross the blood-brain barrier; term coined by Teri Cochrane

Heterozygous

A gene that contains two different alleles—one from the mother and one from the father; one allele is dominant; the other is recessive

High mold food

Food that is naturally susceptible to containing high amounts of mold; these foods are typically peanuts, corn, aged cheeses, certain fruits and vegetables, and other fermented foods

Histamine

An amine that is produced as part of a local immune response and causes inflammation; histamine also performs several important functions in the bowel, and it can act as a neurotransmitter or chemical messenger that carries signals from one nerve to another

Homeostasis

The process through which a variable in the body, like concentration of a certain substance or body temperature, is regulated by the body to remain within a normal range

Homozygous

Two identical forms of a particular gene, one inherited from each parent

Hormonal surge

Occurs when the body increases the level of a certain hormone; for example, women typically experience a hormonal surge of estradiol while ovulating

Hormone imbalance

Occurs when hormones are no longer in balance with each other

Hyperacidity

A chronic condition in which there is an excess of acid in gastric juice, causing discomfort

Hypoglycemia (low blood glucose, low blood sugar)

A condition that occurs when the level of glucose in the blood drops below normal; mild hypoglycemia can cause shakiness, dizziness, lightheadedness, or anxiety; severe hypoglycemia is life threatening

Hypothyroidism

A condition in which an insufficient amount of active thyroid hormone is available in the body; reasons can vary, and include insufficient production in the gland itself, a miscommunication between the brain and the endocrine system, or improper conversion into the active form; symptoms can include lethargy, drier skin, forgetfulness, feeling cold, and constipation

Hypochlorhydria

A state where the production of hydrochloric acid in gastric secretions of the stomach and other digestive organs is absent or lower than needed for optimal function

Impaired detoxification pathway

A buildup of toxins or other metabolic waste products within the body, which can result from increased exposure or burden, or when detoxification-related genes are improperly expressed

Idiopathic

Arising spontaneously from an unknown cause; a word that usually pertains to a disease for which the cause is unknown

Inflammation

A process by which the body's white blood cells, and substances they produce, protect the body from infection or other unfavorable events; short-term inflammation is an appropriate response to injury or a pathogen, but chronic inflammation has been identified as a cause of many modern diseases

Insulin

A hormone created in the pancreas that balances blood glucose levels by allowing the cells and body to absorb glucose and use it as energy; when there is too much glucose in the blood, insulin signals the body to store the extra glucose, which is not released until glucose levels drop below normal; in Type 2 diabetes, the body's cells can become resistant to the action of insulin, resulting in higher blood glucose levels

Intestinal integrity

The degree of intactness of the intestine in maintaining its structure and function, especially in preserving an appropriate barrier between the inside of the digestive tract and the rest of the body

Juicing

The process of extracting the juice from fruits of vegetables, creating a high-nutrient drink

Leaky gut

A condition of increased intestinal permeability or intestinal hyperpermeability in the gut; tight junctions in the gut control what passes through the lining of the small intestine; when these junctions do not work properly, inappropriate substances such as pathogens or undigested food may leak into the bloodstream

Low immunity

When the immune system is poor and does not function properly, therefore causing a person to get sick often or suffer from chronic conditions

Lymphatic system

A part of the circulatory system and a vital part of the immune system, comprising a network of lymphatic vessels that carry a clear fluid called lymph toward the heart; its secondary function is the absorption of fats and fat-soluble vitamins

Malabsorption

A condition that prevents or disrupts absorption of nutrients through the small intestine

Metabolism

The chemical processes that occur within a living organism to maintain life

Methylation

A process by which methyl groups are added to substrates or DNA molecules, facilitating biochemical processes in the body

Microorganism

An organism so small that it cannot be seen with the naked eye; typically a bacterium, virus, or fungus

Mineral

An essential nutrient that the body needs but cannot produce on its own; a balanced diet can provide essential minerals and trace minerals, which are required in smaller amounts

Mold

A fungus that grows indoors or outdoors, usually in damp or moist areas; mold can cause allergic reactions in people who are exposed to large amounts, and in some cases, can cause more significant health risks

Mold spore

Small pollen grain on which mold reproduces itself; spores can travel through the air and be inhaled into the lungs, causing an allergic reaction or asthma attack

Mononucleosis

An infection also known as "mono," which is caused by the Epstein-Barr virus or the Cytomegalovirus and is characterized by fatigue, fever, rash, and swollen glands; it is easily transmitted between individuals through saliva

Mucin

A glycoprotein constituent of mucus that is present in a layer in the digestive tract as well as other organs in the body

Mycotoxin

Toxic secondary metabolites produced by fungus

Myelin

A fatty white substance that surrounds the axon of some nerve cells, forming an electrically insulating layer; myelin is damaged in some neurological diseases

Neuroprotective

Serving to protect nerve cells against damage, degeneration, or impairment of function

Neurotransmitter

A chemical messenger that facilitates communication throughout the nervous system

Non-methylated vitamin

A vitamin that does not contain methyl groups, typically relevant to different forms of B vitamins; these vitamins can be chemically unusable or even harmful to individuals who are unable to metabolize unmethylated forms of certain B vitamins, like folic acid and B12

Nutrient dense

The proportion of nutrients in foods; terms such as nutrient rich and micronutrient dense refer to similar properties

Nutrient

A substance that provides nourishment essential for growth and the maintenance of life

Nutrigenetics

The study of how individual genetic variation affects the absorption of nutrients in the body; it is aimed at optimizing nutrition, health, and disease prevention

Oxalate

Naturally occurring substance found in a wide variety of foods; oxalates play a supportive role in metabolism. In the presence of certain conditions, such as candida, some people may need to remove dietary oxalates from their diet

Oxalate metabolism

The ability to process and metabolize oxalates

Pathogen

Bacterium, virus, or other microorganism that can cause disease

Pathogenic load

A presence of bacteria, viruses, or other microorganisms, which can remain in the body for years after infection; this load can be present even if one is not experiencing symptoms

Pea protein

A vegan, non-dairy type of protein made from the green or yellow pea plant

Peanut

A moldy type of legume that is susceptible to hazardous contaminants and toxins

Permeability

The state of a membrane or barrier that allows certain molecules or substances to pass through it

Polycystic ovary syndrome (PCOS)

A hormonal disorder that may cause small cysts to grow on the ovaries; this disorder can increase a woman's risk for developing insulin resistance, Type 2 diabetes, high cholesterol, high blood pressure, and heart disease; PCOS is often associated with infertility

Polymorphism

Typically used to describe different forms of genes and genetic variation

Polyunsaturated

An organic fat or oil compound that contains several double or triple bonds between the carbon atoms; describes a fat with a more complex structure, making it more vulnerable to damage and oxidation

Probiotics

Supplements containing good or helpful bacteria that are beneficial for the digestive system and general health; often included in food

Protein malabsorption

A state where the body cannot properly break down and use the proteins ingested through food

Protein metabolism

The set biochemical processes through which the body breaks down protein foods into amino acids, which are then recombined to make tissue proteins, tendons, hormones and other necessary elements for the body

Protein size

How small or large a protein molecule is based on the number of amino acids that make up the protein chain

Protocol

An official procedure or set of rules designed for a specific purpose

Proton-pump inhibitor (PPI)

A class of medications used for reduction of gastric acid production

Psoriasis

A disease mediated by the immune system and genetics, which causes raised, red, scaly patches to appear on the skin

Rheumatoid arthritis (RA)

An autoimmune disease caused by inflammation and characterized by pain, swelling, and stiffness of the joints, as well as fatigue and muscle pain

Root cause

The origin of a condition or the initiation of a causal chain

Selectively permeable cell membrane

A cell membrane that allows only certain molecules or ions to pass through

Sensitivity

When the body has trouble breaking down specific types of molecules due to an issue within a certain pathway in the body; for example, those who have a sulfur sensitivity have trouble breaking down and using sulfur, because their sulfur pathways are not optimally functional

Soaking

The act of wetting something thoroughly; typically accomplished by leaving a legume, seed or nut in a glass container in a small amount of water overnight

Sprouting

The process of germinating seeds, grains, or beans that are to be eaten

Staphylococcus (staph)

A group of bacteria that most commonly causes skin infections in the form of red, swollen boils on the skin; can cause infections like pneumonia, food poisoning, toxic shock syndrome, and others

Starch

A polymeric carbohydrate made up of many glucose units; starch is produced by most green plants as an energy store; it is common in the human diet, and it is found in high amounts in food like potatoes, wheat, and rice

Stool

The solid waste of the human digestive system; stool varies in appearance based on digestive system health, diet, and general health

Streptococcus (strep)

A bacteria that causes an infection such as strep throat; symptoms of strep throat typically include a red, sore throat, swollen tonsils, and white spots in the throat; this bacteria can remain in the body for a long time after exposure, even without producing symptoms

Sulfate

Any chemical compounds related to sulfuric acid; sulfate is usually a desirable end product of sulfur metabolism in the body

Sulfur

A compound on the periodic table that is a necessary part of a healthy diet; it is found in higher concentration in certain foods such as cruciferous vegetables and eggs; for some people, excessive ingestion of sulfur-rich foods can cause negative symptoms and contribute to dysfunction

Sulfur metabolism

The biochemical process by which the body breaks down sulfur to make sulfur-containing compounds that help the body function properly

Sugar

The generic name for sweet, soluble carbohydrates, many of which are used in food

SUOX

A gene that is an important component of the sulfur pathway in the body; enzymes produced by this gene are used to convert sulfite into sulfate

Symptomatic

The state of exhibiting a symptom of a particular disease or condition

The *Tru of You*™

A term for finding your individual truth to help reach optimal health and wellbeing; term coined by Teri Cochrane

Thyroid stimulating hormone (TSH)

A hormone that causes the thyroid gland to produce T3 and T4, which are two hormones that help regulate metabolism and many other key processes in the body

Tight junction

Junctions that serve to seal the space where two adjacent epithelial cells meet, blocking the passage of undesirable molecules and ions; this most often refers to the space between epithelial cells in the gut and is desirable to prevent disease; see leaky gut

Tipping point

The point at which the body can no longer manage multiple metabolic processes without becoming symptomatic

Toxic load

A load in the body, potentially harmful to a person's health, that is formed by the toxins and chemicals that a person is exposed to through processed foods, the surrounding environment, and stress

Ulcerative colitis (UC)

A chronic disease in which the lining of the colon becomes inflamed, causing the formation of tiny open sore (ulcers) that produce pus and mucous; symptoms can include abdominal pain, loose and bloody stools, and persistent diarrhea

Wild meats

Meats less likely to contain amyloids, usually those that are not commercially processed in the United States

Wildatarian™ Type

The type of **Wildatarian** diet plan best suited for your body and its genetics; these types include **W–TYPE Wildatarian** Basic, **WF–TYPE Wildatarian** (Low-Fat), **WS–TYPE Wildatarian** (Low-Sulfur), and **WSF–TYPE Wildatarian** (Low-Fat and Low-Sulfur;) terms coined by Teri Cochrane

Yeast

An organism that helps with digestion and nutrient absorption; candida, a species of yeast, is present mainly in small amounts in the mouth and intestines; however, the body can also experience yeast overgrowth, which can cause problems like a leaky gut; yeast overgrowth can express as yeast infections, nail fungus, fungal rashes, and dandruff.

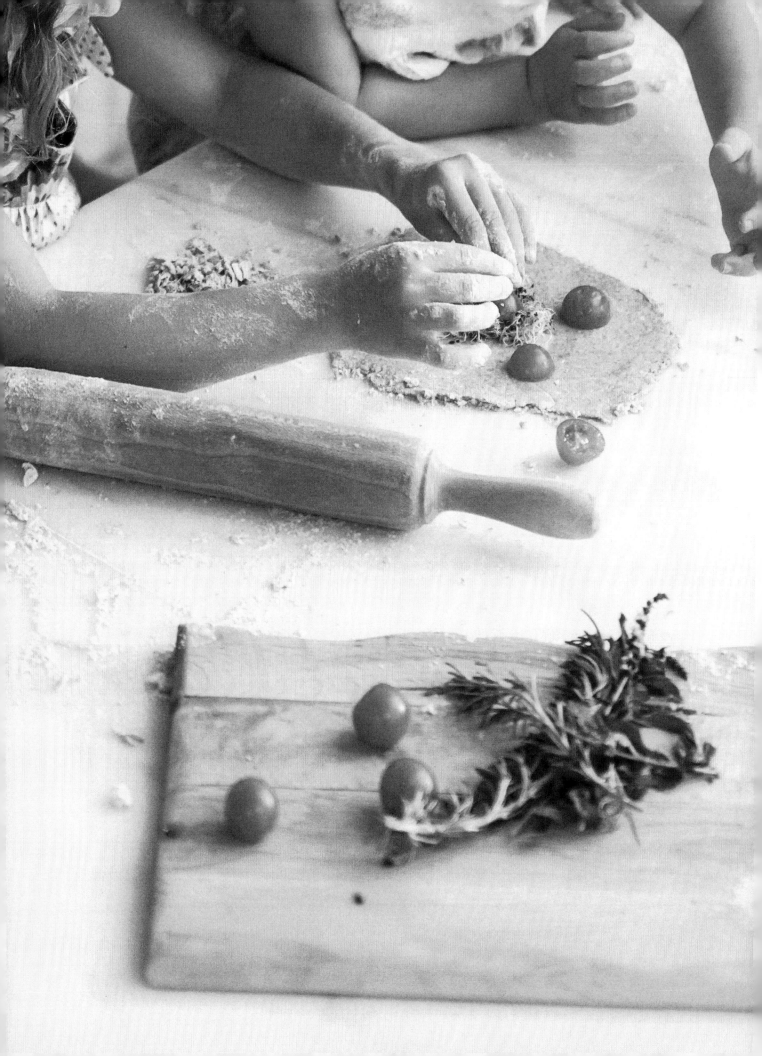

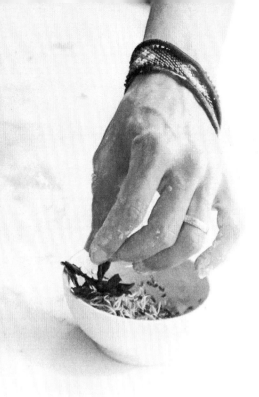

WILDATARIAN RECIPES

ANDALUSIAN SNAPPER

SERVES 4

I build a renewed system free of toxins and waste with this full-flavored meal.

Drawing its inspiration from the sultry southern part of Spain, this flavorful dish features snapper, a favorite fish in Spanish cooking. Snapper is an excellent source of omega-3 fatty acids and selenium—a mineral needed for the proper functioning of our antioxidant system. Selenium is a precursor of glutathione peroxidase, one of the most important antioxidants, which supports the elimination of toxic waste from our cells and body. Consumption of selenium and omega-3 rich foods has been associated with a decreased risk of colon cancer. There are synergistic effects when taking in selenium with vitamins C, E, and A. Tomatoes are a rich source of vitamin C, and by pairing this recipe with roasted plantains and fresh cilantro, you also gain the benefits of vitamin A and potassium. Fresh cilantro is a wonderful kidney detoxifier and works synergistically with the snapper to aid in detoxification.

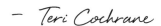

— *Teri Cochrane*

- 2 medium sweet onions, sliced into rings
- ¼ cup Spanish olive oil
- 4 red snapper fillets
- ¼ cup white wine
- ½ cup black olives, cut into rounds
- One 16-ounce can diced tomatoes
- Dash of sea salt
- ⅛ teaspoon freshly ground pepper
- ½ cup chopped fresh parsley
- 2 cups cooked brown rice, brown rice pasta, or quinoa

In a large cast iron skillet over medium heat, sauté onions in olive oil until semi-tender, about 5 minutes. Add red snapper fillets, white wine, olives, diced tomatoes, and salt and pepper. Mix well and cook until liquid is absorbed and fish is white and flaky, about 3 to 5 minutes. Add parsley a minute or two before removing pan from the stove. Serve over brown rice, brown rice pasta, or quinoa.

APPLICABILITY TO FOOD PLANS

W	Follow recipe as is	WF	Follow recipe as is
WS	Reduce amount of onions specified by half and cook them thoroughly	WFS	Reduce amount of onions specified by half and cook them thoroughly

AVOCADO, PAPAYA, AND CILANTRO SALAD

SERVES 4

Potassium keeps my muscles moving and my heart strong; I am grateful.

The avocado, papaya, and cilantro in this recipe display magnificent colors, and together they are a potassium powerhouse. Potassium is important in regulating heart function, reducing blood pressure, and converting glucose into glycogen for use by our muscles. It also is a pH balancer. Serve this salad as an appetizer or as a side dish with beans, wild game, or fish.

— Teri Cochrane

- 2 avocados, peeled, pitted, and cut into cubes
- 2 cups fresh papaya, peeled, pitted, and cut into cubes
- 1 cup coarsely chopped fresh cilantro
- Freshly squeezed juice from ½ lime
- ½ teaspoon sea salt

Combine all ingredients in a serving bowl. Toss together and chill for 5 to 10 minutes.

*Note: During the **Maintenance** phase, you may substitute mango for papaya.*

APPLICABILITY TO FOOD PLANS

W	Follow recipe as is	**WF**	Follow recipe as is
WS	Follow recipe as is	**WFS**	Follow recipe as is

AVOCADO, TOMATO, AND HUMMUS WRAP

SERVES 1

Cool and crisp flavors supply me with beneficial oils and proteins.

This is one of my favorite wraps when I am traveling. I put the ingredients in a cooler, and at lunch time, I just wrap and roll! Assembling ingredients is all that is necessary; there is no need to turn on your oven or stove top, nor to make the "drive of shame" (as coined by one of my clients) to a fast food establishment. The avocado provides good fats and oils and helps to metabolize excess estrogen in the body. Hummus is a protein source; the tomatoes supply ample antioxidants; and the cucumbers are a cooling vegetable, rich in silica, which supports healthy, hair, bones, and tissue.

— *Teri Cochrane*

- ½ small California avocado, peeled and pitted
- ½ teaspoon extra virgin olive oil
- 2 tablespoons hummus
- 1 gluten-free whole grain tortilla
- 4 slices cucumber
- 4 to 6 grape tomatoes, halved
- Sea salt
- Freshly ground black pepper

In a medium bowl, mash avocado; mix with olive oil. Spread avocado and hummus evenly on the tortilla. Top with cucumber slices and tomato halves. Season with salt and pepper to taste. Roll the wrap into a cylinder, and serve with fresh fruit or salad greens.

As a variation, you can add ½ cup grilled **Herb-Rubbed Roasted Duck** breast (page 128), **Wild Boar Carnitas** (page 150), or any other **Wildatarian** protein source, and assemble as directed above.

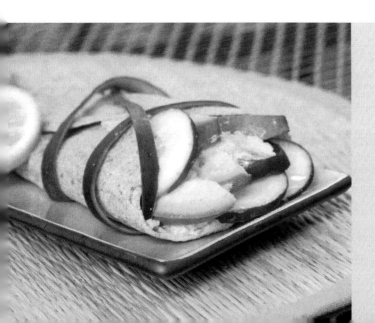

APPLICABILITY TO FOOD PLANS

W	Follow recipe as is
WS	Use a hummus that does not contain garlic
WF	Follow recipe as is
WFS	Use a hummus that does not contain garlic

BANANA, BUCKWHEAT, AND CHOCOLATE CHIP MUFFINS

MAKES 12 MUFFINS

My stomach is soothed, and I find new strength and energy with every bite.

I love buckwheat because it is high in fiber like oats and is a complete, easily digestible, gluten-free protein like quinoa. Cream of buckwheat is a good alternative to oatmeal and can be found at most health food grocers. Although categorized as a grain, buckwheat is a fruit seed that is related to rhubarb and sorrel. Buckwheat flour has a hint of purple in its color, so these muffins will look pretty and be pretty tasty. This is such a protein-packed muffin that I have added in a little chocolate for good measure.

— *Teri Cochrane*

- 1 large egg, beaten
- 1½ cups unsweetened goat milk, coconut or almond milk beverage
- ⅓ cup honey
- 1 overripe banana, mashed
- 4 ounces natural applesauce
- 1 teaspoon vanilla extract
- 1⅓ cup buckwheat flour
- 1½ cup quinoa flour
- 1⅓ tablespoon aluminum-free baking powder
- ½ teaspoon cinnamon
- ½ teaspoon sea salt
- 2 tablespoons turbinado or organic natural cane sugar
- ½ cup semisweet chocolate chips

Preheat oven to 350°F. Place 12 muffin liners into a standard 2 ½-inch diameter muffin tray that holds approximately ¼ cup batter per muffin. In a large mixing bowl, place egg, milk, honey, banana, applesauce, and vanilla; stir to combine. Beat dry ingredients (buckwheat flour, quinoa flour, baking powder, cinnamon, sea salt, and sugar) into liquids until well combined. Fold in chocolate chips. Divide batter evenly among liners. Bake for approximately 25 minutes until toothpick comes out clean.

Note: Although egg yolks contain sulfur, this recipe is safe for WS and WSF because one egg is distributed across 12 muffins.

APPLICABILITY TO FOOD PLANS

W	Not appropriate for the **Rebalance** phase
WS	Not appropriate for the **Rebalance** phase
WF	Not appropriate for the **Rebalance** phase
WFS	Not appropriate for the **Rebalance** phase

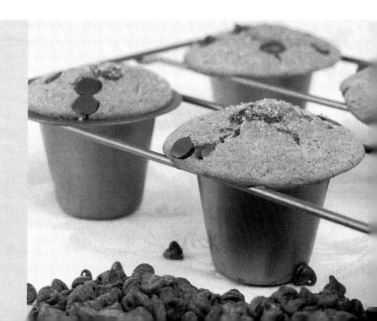

BERRYFUL STEEL-CUT OATMEAL

I choose optimal health for my body and my soul each morning.

The picture featured for this recipe is my message to you that you hold your health in your hands. Breakfast is truly the most important meal. It is essential that you eat breakfast every day, but it is even more important that you choose your breakfast foods wisely. The "Second Meal Effect" explains that the benefits, or lack thereof, of the food we eat at breakfast carry over into our second meal of the day.

Starting your day with steel-cut oatmeal, in any of the variations offered, will help to balance your blood sugar levels. This meal also will provide fiber from the oatmeal for easier evacuation (which aids in detoxification), antioxidants from our berry friends, and simple proteins and essential fatty acids from the many varieties of nuts. The "Berryful" version will only get tastier if you make extra and save it for future breakfasts. The berry flavors are infused further into the oatmeal each day. Do not store longer than four days.

— Teri Cochrane

- 4 cups filtered water
- ½ teaspoon salt
- 1 cup steel cut oats
- ½ cup dried sulfite-free cherries
- ½ cup dried sulfite-free wild blueberries

Prepare basic oatmeal: bring water and salt to a boil in a medium saucepan. Add oats and lower heat to a simmer. Cook approximately 30 to 35 minutes; stir occasionally and allow oats to reach a creamy consistency. About 10 minutes before the oatmeal is done, fold in cherries and blueberries. Continue cooking, stirring occasionally to prevent the oatmeal from sticking to the bottom of the pan. Add additional water by the tablespoon, as necessary, to achieve desired consistency. Serve with non-dairy milk, such as coconut or almond milk.

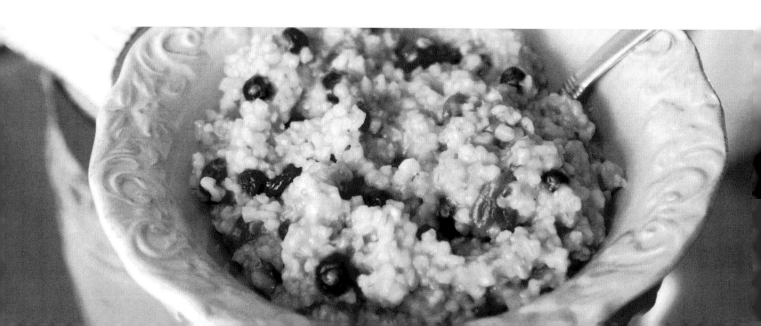

Here are some variations for this recipe to be used during the **Maintenance** Phase:

- **Coconut Pineapple Mango:** Prepare basic oatmeal using one cup lite canned coconut milk with 3 cups of water. Top with fresh mango and pineapple chunks.

- **Fresh Papaya and Pumpkin Seed:** Prepare basic oatmeal. Top with fresh papaya, pumpkin seeds and honey.

- **Nutty Delight:** Prepare basic oatmeal. Five minutes before removing from stove, stir in chopped almonds, sunflower seeds, and 1 teaspoon of ground flaxseed. Top with honey. Skip this version if you are a WF or WFS.

APPLICABILITY TO FOOD PLANS

W	Not appropriate for the **Rebalance** phase		**WF**	Not appropriate for the **Rebalance** phase
WS	Not appropriate for the **Rebalance** phase		**WFS**	Not appropriate for the **Rebalance** phase

BLACK BEAN DIP

These turtle beans support my blood sugar and mood, and I am satisfied.

This simple-to-make dip is a crowd pleaser, whether you are hosting a fancy dinner party or tailgating at a football game. Best of all, it is chock-full of fiber and plant-based protein.

— Teri Cochrane

- 2 cups Cuban black beans, at room temperature
- 1 cup mild chunky salsa
- 1 tablespoon lime juice
- ¼ teaspoon salt
- ¼ teaspoon cracked pepper
- ¼ teaspoon cumin

Combine all ingredients in a large bowl. Serve with organic blue corn or other gluten-free multigrain chips.

This dip also can be:

• served puréed.

• heated with one cup filtered water and served as a soup with a dollop of goat yogurt and chopped green onion as a topping.

• spread on a tortilla and topped with tomato, avocado, and cilantro for an easy burrito lunch option.

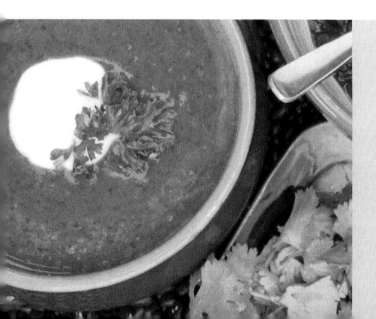

APPLICABILITY TO FOOD PLANS

W	Follow recipe as is
WS	Reduce salsa by half in **Rebalance** phase
WF	Follow recipe as is
WFS	Reduce salsa by half in **Rebalance** phase

BYOJ (BUILD YOUR OWN JUICE)

By sipping in chlorophyll, phytonutrients, and antioxidants, I am restored.

Juicing first thing in the morning is a great way to support healthy pH balance and boost immunity. Different juice combinations can be mixed and matched. These juices will help wake you up, as they are abundant in chlorophyll, alkalizing agents, phytonutrients, antioxidants, minerals, and vitamins, and such vibrant colors. Once you make juicing a morning habit, you will notice a positive difference in the way you feel.

— *Teri Cochrane*

Juice Base:

- ½ regular or English cucumber

Optional Add-Ins (Rule of thumb: three vegetables to one fruit):

- 1 cup fresh cilantro, rinsed
- 4 stalks celery, rinsed
- 1 cup fresh parsley, rinsed
- 4 Swiss chard leaves, rinsed
- 3 beet tops, rinsed
- 1 beetroot
- ½ lime or lemon, peeled
- 1 inch ginger root
- 1 cup spinach leaves, rinsed

- 1 cup strawberries, rinsed
- ¼ cabbage, chunked
- 1 cup watermelon, rind removed, chunked
- 1 carrot, chunked

Wash, peel, and juice cucumber. To create your unique morning juice, add any or all of the above add-ins with the cucumber. Mix and drink at once or sip throughout the day. Although not optimal, juice can be refrigerated in a glass container such as a mason jar for up to three days.

A serving is 4 ounces of juice mixed with 8 ounces of water.

APPLICABILITY TO FOOD PLANS

W	Follow recipe as is
WS	Eliminate cabbage and celery as juice ingredients
WF	Eliminate carrots as juice ingredient in **Rebalance** phase
WFS	Eliminate cabbage and celery as juice ingredients Eliminate carrots as juice ingredient in **Rebalance** phase

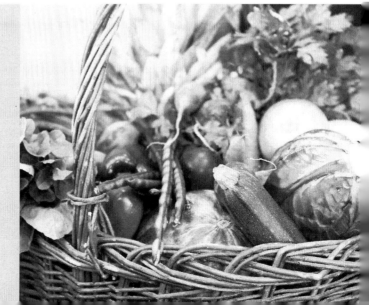

CHINESE WILD SHRIMP AND CABBAGE

As I eat this powerfully beneficial dish, I feel youthful and fresh.

Cooking the veggies until just tender gives this recipe a really fresh flavor. Combined, these vegetables contain pure and excellent forms of vitamins A, C, and K in addition to an assortment of minerals including calcium, iron, and manganese. The greens are also potent liver purifiers. Bean sprouts have been touted to have anti-aging effects. Shrimp is an easily digested protein full of minerals from the sea.

— Teri Cochrane

- 4 tablespoons olive oil
- 1 medium onion, cut into large chunks
- 2 pounds peeled and deveined wild shrimp
- ¼ teaspoon salt
- ¼ cup honey
- ¼ cup tamari sauce
- 4 medium carrots, cut into thin strips
- ½ head of cabbage, rinsed and cut into strips
- 4 medium collard leaves, rinsed, tough ribs removed, and cut in crosswise strips
- 1 cup fresh bean sprouts, rinsed (optional)

In large skillet or wok, heat olive oil, and stir-fry onions, shrimp, and salt over high heat for about 4 to 6 minutes, until the shrimp is almost fully cooked. Remove shrimp and onions from skillet and set aside in a bowl. Heat honey, tamari sauce, and carrots in skillet. Stir-fry about 3 minutes until carrots are tender. Add cabbage, and stir-fry an additional 2 to 3 minutes, until just tender. Add collards, and continue stir-frying for 1 to 2 minutes. Return shrimp to skillet and lower to medium heat; cook 1 to 2 minutes. Add bean sprouts to warm them, but do not overcook. Serve over brown basmati rice.

APPLICABILITY TO FOOD PLANS

W Eliminate honey in **Rebalance** phase

WS Eliminate honey in **Rebalance** phase
Substitute zucchini or yellow squash for cabbage
Substitute spinach for collards
Reduce amount of onions by 50% and cook thoroughly in **Rebalance** phase

WF Eliminate honey in **Rebalance** phase
Substitute zucchini or yellow squash for carrots in **Rebalance** phase

WFS Eliminate honey in **Rebalance** phase
Substitute zucchini or yellow squash for cabbage
Substitute spinach for collards
Reduce amount of onions specified by 50% and cook thoroughly in **Rebalance** phase

CINNAMON OAT PANCAKES

I enjoy good digestion from this fiber and these protective spices.

This tasty, wheat-free pancake is high in fiber and low in sugar, and contains healthy fats from the nut milks. Standard pancakes are filled with refined ingredients, which makes digestion difficult. The combination of cinnamon and honey offers a synergistic effect, because when consumed together, they spark immunity, improve digestion, help to reduce cholesterol, and improve heart health.

— *Teri Cochrane*

- 1 cup oat flour
- 1 tablespoon aluminum-free baking powder
- ¾ teaspoon sea salt
- 1 teaspoon cinnamon
- 1 cup unsweetened coconut or almond beverage
- 4 ounces unsweetened plain or naturally flavored applesauce
- 1 teaspoon vanilla extract
- 1 large egg, beaten
- Honey, or fresh seasonal fruit, coconut, or monk fruit sugar for serving

Heat electric griddle to 375°F or place large skillet over medium heat. In a medium bowl, stir together flour, baking powder, salt, and cinnamon. In a small bowl, mix milk, applesauce, vanilla, and egg, and add to dry ingredients. Beat until combined well. Dip ¼ measuring cup into batter and pour onto greased hot griddle or skillet. Cook on one side until bubbles form around the edges. Turn, and cook until fluffy and cooked thoroughly. Top with honey, fresh fruit, coconut, or monk fruit sugar.

APPLICABILITY TO FOOD PLANS

W	Not appropriate for the **Rebalance** phase
WS	Not appropriate for the **Rebalance** phase
WF	Not appropriate for the **Rebalance** phase
WFS	Not appropriate for the **Rebalance** phase

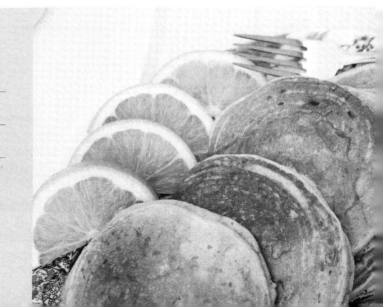

COCONUT ARROZ CON LECHE

SERVES 6

I enjoy this rich-tasting treat, knowing that I am protected from unhealthy sugars.

In this sweet treat, I have replaced the white arborio rice commonly used in Spanish rice pudding recipes with a short grain brown rice, which looks like its chubby, refined cousin, but provides B vitamins, magnesium, and fiber. Coconut milk takes the place of dairy. The coconut milk contains lauric acid, which has antimicrobial, antiviral, and antifungal properties. Who knew coconut milk could be so healthful? The liberal use of cinnamon in this recipe brings forth multiple health benefits. Seasoning a high carbohydrate food such as this one with cinnamon can help to lessen its impact on blood sugar levels. Cinnamon's essential oils also possess antimicrobial qualities, which may help stop the growth of pathogens including the commonly problematic yeast, candida.

— *Teri Cochrane*

- 1 cup short-grain brown rice
- 4 cups water
- 1 cinnamon stick
- ¼ teaspoon sea salt
- 2 cups canned organic lite coconut milk
- ⅓ cup honey
- 1 cup sulfite-free raisins (optional)
- 1 teaspoon ground cinnamon

Place rice, water, cinnamon stick, and salt in a pressure cooker. Place on high heat until pressure cooker is pressurized; lower heat to medium-low. Cook for 40 minutes and remove from heat. Wait for 5 minutes to allow cooker to depressurize; open lid. Warm the milk and honey in a small pot over low heat, stirring occasionally. Open pressure cooker, remove cinnamon stick from rice and discard. Add milk mixture to rice in cooker. Stir frequently over medium-low heat. Stir in raisins if using. Place rice mixture in 9 by 12-inch glass, ceramic serving dish, or individual serving dishes. Refrigerate for one hour. Top with ground cinnamon and serve.

Note: No pressure cooker? Then, make recipe as instructed but cook water, rice, cinnamon stick, and salt for 60 minutes.

APPLICABILITY TO FOOD PLANS

W Substitute monk fruit sugar for honey in **Rebalance** phase
Eliminate raisins in **Rebalance** phase

WS Substitute monk fruit sugar for honey in **Rebalance** phase
Eliminate raisins in **Rebalance** phase

WF Substitute monk fruit sugar for honey in **Rebalance** phase
Eliminate raisins in **Rebalance** phase
Substitute coconut milk beverage for canned coconut milk

WFS Substitute monk fruit sugar for honey in **Rebalance** phase
Eliminate raisins in **Rebalance** phase
Substitute coconut milk beverage for canned coconut milk

CUBAN BLACK BEANS

I am free and clear of toxins by eating these good-for-me beans every day.

The combination of the dried beans, garlic, and cumin in this recipe is a powerhouse for detoxification. The black beans, like lentils, pack a high fiber punch (15 grams per one cup serving), but black beans also contain a phenomenal amount of the trace mineral molybdenum, which helps to detoxify sulfites. Sulfites are a type of preservative commonly added to prepared foods. This is not good news, as many people, especially those with any neurological dysfunction, are sensitive to sulfites. A cup of black beans will give you almost 200 percent of the daily requirement for this helpful trace mineral. Cumin has been shown to enhance the liver's detoxification enzymes.

— Teri Cochrane

- One 16-ounce bag of dried black beans
- 1 clove garlic, peeled
- ½ onion, cut in quarters
- 1 teaspoon sea salt
- 1 to 2 tablespoons cumin
- 1 teaspoon sea salt
- 1 teaspoon balsamic vinegar
- ½ teaspoon turbinado sugar

In a pressure cooker, place beans, garlic, onion, and salt. Add water to cover beans, so that the pressure cooker is roughly ¾ full. Tightly secure pressure cooker lid. Place over high heat until pressure cooker is pressurized; lower to medium-low heat. Cook for 1½ hours. Remove from heat and allow cooker to depressurize. Open lid. Add cumin, salt, vinegar, and sugar. Mix well. Simmer over medium-low heat for 20 minutes or until desired consistency is reached. Serve with brown or basmati rice.

Note: No pressure cooker? Place 10 cups of filtered water, beans, garlic or onions, and salt in a Dutch oven. Bring to a boil. Reduce heat and simmer over medium heat for 2 to 3 hours, stirring occasionally until beans are tender. Once beans are cooked, follow remaining instructions above.

(continued)

APPLICABILITY TO FOOD PLANS

W	Substitute apple cider vinegar for balsamic vinegar in **Rebalance** phase
WS	Eliminate garlic from recipe Substitute apple cider vinegar for balsamic vinegar in **Rebalance** phase
WF	Substitute apple cider vinegar for balsamic vinegar in **Rebalance** phase
WFS	Eliminate garlic from recipe Substitute apple cider vinegar for balsamic vinegar in **Rebalance** phase

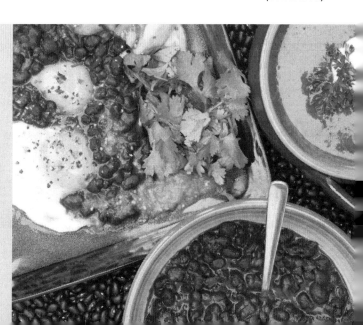

CUBAN BLACK BEANS

(continued)

CONVERTIBLES

Black beans are so versatile that this is one of my favorite recipes for making many more creations with a few simple additions.

BLACK BEAN CARROT SOUP

- 2 cups Cuban Black Beans
- 1 cup water
- 2 cups chopped carrots
- 1 cup chopped fresh cilantro

Mix all ingredients well. Simmer over medium-low heat for 5 minutes.

Serves 2

HUEVOS RANCHEROS

- 4 eggs
- salt and pepper to taste
- 1 avocado, sliced
- 1 cup Cuban Black Beans
- ⅓ cup salsa

In a bowl, crack eggs, and fold until fluffy. Add salt and pepper to taste. In a greased cast iron skillet over medium heat add eggs and scramble to desired state of consistency. Remove from heat. Top scrambled eggs with Cuban black beans and salsa. Serve with avocado slices. This also can be made into a breakfast burrito; just put all of the ingredients in a whole grain, gluten-free tortilla and enjoy!

Serves 2

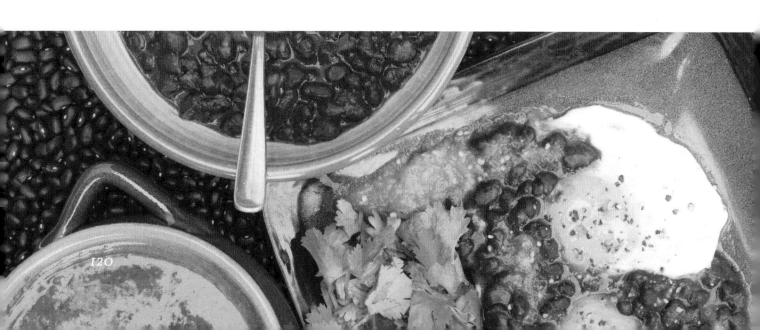

CUBAN ROPA VIEJA

I am renewed when I prepare and partake of this healthful protein.

"Old Clothes," as this dish is called, is my son's all-time favorite. This is a popular Cuban dish, usually made from flank steak, but I use buffalo chuck roast instead. Because of buffalo's high protein content, it tends to be drier than beef. Boiling the buffalo really tenderizes it and yields a broth to use as a base for soup. The flavor that buffalo imparts is smoky and rich. Buffalo is usually raised without hormones or antibiotics, so not only will you be getting a better protein source, but you'll also be avoiding unwanted hormone disruptors and drugs.

— *Teri Cochrane*

For the buffalo:

- 10 cups filtered water
- 2 pounds buffalo (or bison) chuck
- ½ large onion, diced
- 2 cloves garlic, minced
- 1 teaspoon salt

In large stockpot over medium-high heat, bring to a boil buffalo or bison, onion, garlic (as appropriate), and salt. Reduce heat to medium-low, cover and continue cooking until meat is cooked through, approximately 40 minutes. Remove buffalo from broth and shred, using two forks. Set aside. Strain beef broth and store for later use.

For the Ropa Vieja:

- 3 tablespoons olive oil, divided
- 4 cloves garlic, minced
- 1 large onion, diced
- 1 diced green bell pepper, seeds and ribs removed
- 3 ounces tomato paste
- 3 ounces water
- ¼ teaspoon freshly ground black pepper
- One 8-ounce can tomato sauce
- 1 teaspoon ground cumin
- 1 teaspoon dried oregano
- 2 medium bay leaves

APPLICABILITY TO FOOD PLANS

W	Follow recipe as is	WF	Follow recipe as is
WS	Eliminate garlic from recipe	WFS	Eliminate garlic from recipe

CUBAN ROPA VIEJA

(continued)

For the Ropa Vieja:

Heat 2 tablespoon olive oil in skillet on medium heat. Stir in garlic (as appropriate), onion, and green bell pepper, and cook until onions are translucent, about 3 to 5 minutes. Dilute tomato paste with water. Stir in black pepper, buffalo, tomato sauce, diluted tomato paste, cumin, oregano, and bay leaves. Cook for an additional 15 minutes to infuse flavors. Serve on top of brown rice.

CONVERTIBLE

BUFFALO QUINOA VEGETABLE SOUP
(This is a play on beef and barley soup)

- 6 to 8 cups buffalo broth
- ½ cup quinoa
- 12 ounce bag of frozen vegetables, thawed
- 14 ounce can undrained, diced, fire roasted tomatoes
- 1 teaspoon dried oregano
- ½ teaspoon salt
- ¼ teaspoon freshly ground black pepper

In a stockpot, add buffalo broth, quinoa, vegetables, fire roasted tomatoes, dried oregano, salt, and freshly ground black pepper. Bring the soup to a boil. Reduce heat to a simmer, and cook for 20 minutes. For WS, or WFS, use non-sulfur frozen vegetables.

Serves 6 to 8

CURRIED LENTILS WITH WILD RICE

SERVES 6

Mighty lentils fuel me with healthful protein and fiber.

Lentils, mighty little members of the legume family, are a great source of dietary fiber, iron, and protein. Just one cup provides 16 grams of fiber, which is about half of the recommended daily serving. These little guys also help with stabilizing blood sugar levels and provide anti-inflammatory benefits. Lentils are a wonderful protein and iron source for vegetarians, and pairing them with wild rice, as in this recipe, provides a complete protein. Additionally, lentils are rich in folate, which helps lower levels of homocysteine, an amino acid that has been linked to cardiovascular disease and other inflammatory conditions.

— *Teri Cochrane*

- One 16-ounce bag dried lentils
- 8 cups filtered water
- 1 medium onion, cut into quarters
- 1 teaspoon ground cumin
- 1 teaspoon ground curry powder
- ¼ teaspoon ground cinnamon
- 2 teaspoons sea salt
- 2 cups wild rice

Place the lentils, water, and onion in a stock pot over medium-high heat. Cover and cook for 30 to 45 minutes or until lentils are tender, stirring occasionally. Mix in cumin, curry, cinnamon, and salt. Cook until desired consistency is achieved, approximately 10 minutes, stirring occasionally to prevent burning. Prepare the wild rice according to package instructions. Serve the lentils over the wild rice.

APPLICABILITY TO FOOD PLANS

W	Follow recipe as is
WS	Reduce amount of onions specified in half and cook thoroughly
WF	Follow recipe as is
WFS	Reduce amount of onions specified in half and cook thoroughly

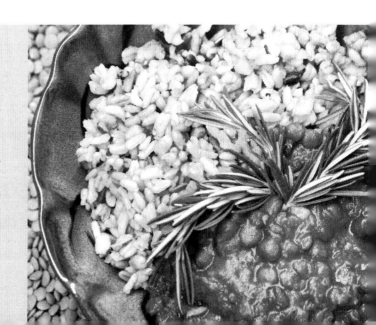

DUCK PAELLA

I know who I am and how my soul is fed with these healthful fats and heart-protective vegetables.

I have been eating some form of paella since I was a little girl. This dish, although more complicated than most of my other recipes, is so worth the extra effort. Replacing the Valencia rice with short brown rice provides a whole grain and is beautifully suited as a healthier substitute. Using duck provides a rich flavor with amazing fats. If you have leftovers from this dish, they will taste even better the next day, as the flavors continue to enhance each other.

— Teri Cochrane

- 4 boneless, skinless duck breasts
- 2 boneless, skinless duck thighs
- ½ green pepper, chopped with seeds and ribs removed
- 1 red pepper, ½ chopped, ½ sliced with seeds and ribs removed
- ½ medium onion, chopped
- 3 cloves garlic, minced
- 1 teaspoon sea salt, divided in half
- 2 tablespoons olive oil
- 5 cups short-grain brown rice
- 5½ cups filtered water
- One 14-ounce can fire roasted tomatoes, diced
- One 6-ounce can tomato sauce
- 2 bay leaves
- 1 teaspoon oregano
- 1 cup roasted red pepper

In a Dutch oven over medium heat, sauté the duck, chopped green and red peppers, onion, garlic, and ½ teaspoon salt in the olive oil, until duck is browned, about 5 minutes. In pressure cooker, place rice, water, tomatoes, tomato sauce, bay leaves, oregano, and remaining salt. Add duck and vegetable mixture. Place on high heat until pressure cooker is pressurized; reduce to medium-low heat. Cook for 40 minutes; remove from heat. Allow cooker to depressurize; open lid. Return all ingredients to Dutch oven. On low heat, cook until rice is of desired consistency and water has been further absorbed, about 15 minutes. Spoon onto serving platter. Top with roasted red pepper slices.

Note: No pressure cooker? Cook duck and vegetable mixture per instructions, then place all of the ingredients in a large cooking pot. Bring to a boil, then cover and reduce to a simmer. Cook for 1 hour and 10 minutes, stirring occasionally.

APPLICABILITY TO FOOD PLANS

W	Follow recipe as is	**WF**	Not appropriate for the **Rebalance** phase Only use duck breast in **Maintenance** phase
WS	Eliminate garlic from recipe	**WFS**	Not appropriate for the **Rebalance** phase Only use duck breast in **Maintenance** phase

FRUIT AND NUT BREAD PUDDING

SERVES 8

Sweet fruit and nuts satiate me while replenishing my body with energizing fuel.

Oh, the horror of refined carbohydrates, trans fats, and sugar in traditional bread pudding—well, not in this version! The traditional refined white bread has been replaced with a gluten-free, whole-grain alternative, and the nuts and coconut milk give it a nice, light consistency. The whole grains and fats from the coconut milk help slow the sugar absorption into the bloodstream, and sulfite-free dried fruit lends natural sweetness. This dairy- and wheat-free version is a great treat for people with those sensitivities, and no substituting flavor: it is wonderfully tasty.

— *Teri Cochrane*

- 2 cups almond milk
- 1 cup lite canned coconut milk
- ⅔ cup honey
- 2 tablespoons organic butter
- 3 large eggs
- 1 teaspoon cinnamon
- 2 teaspoons vanilla extract
- 4 cups whole grain gluten-free bread, cut into cubes
- ⅓ cup raw, coarsely chopped almonds
- ⅓ cup raw cashews
- ⅓ cup sulfite-free raisins
- ⅓ cup sulfite-free dried cranberries or cherries

Preheat oven to 350°F. Grease a 9 by 13-inch glass or ceramic baking dish. In a 3 to 4-quart saucepan, add milk, honey, and butter. Warm the milk mixture over low heat, stirring occasionally until butter melts. In a large mixing bowl, whisk together eggs, cinnamon, and vanilla. Slowly add milk mixture to the eggs, whisking constantly until completely blended. Place bread in prepared baking dish. Pour liquid mixture over bread, making sure bread is completely moistened. Fold nuts, raisins, and cranberries into bread mixture. Bake in oven for 40 to 50 minutes or until a knife inserted in the center of the casserole comes out clean and the bread is browned. Serve warm.

Note: Even if you have a sulfur sensitivity, it is fine to bake with whole eggs.

APPLICABILITY TO FOOD PLANS

W	Not appropriate for the **Rebalance** phase	**WF**	Not appropriate for the **Rebalance** phase
WS	Not appropriate for the **Rebalance** phase	**WFS**	Not appropriate for the **Rebalance** phase

GREEN GARDEN SOUP

SERVES 8

I am energized by these deep greens from nature's garden as my body receives rich oxygen from the chlorophyll.

I recommend using the soup to break your nighttime fast during the cold winter months. This is a great choice for getting your fill of greens and chlorophyll; the veggies are rich in antioxidants and chemical compounds known for inhibiting cancer cell growth. All of the greens in this soup are great liver detoxifiers and alkalizers. Using the medicinal herbs adds more health benefits so that your cup of healthful soup overfloweth. Serving this soup with a fresh squeeze of lime brings out the flavors of the greens. Use bone broth to add protein; add beans to increase fiber.

— Teri Cochrane

- 8 cups filtered water or bone broth
- 1 large onion, chopped
- One 12-ounce bag fresh spinach
- 1 cup chopped fresh parsley
- 2 cups broccoli florets
- ½ head cabbage, chopped
- 5 medium collard leaves, tough ribs removed, cut in crosswise strips
- 2 cups peeled, chopped sweet potato
- 1 to 2 teaspoons sea salt
- Freshly ground black pepper
- 1 teaspoon dried oregano
- ¼ teaspoon dried basil (optional)

- 2 cups any type of cooked or canned beans, rinsed and drained
- 1 lime, cut into 8 wedges

In a large pot over high heat, add water or bone broth and remaining ingredients except the lime; bring to a boil. Reduce heat to simmer, stirring occasionally. Cook until vegetables are tender, roughly 45 minutes to 1 hour. Serve with lime wedges.

APPLICABILITY TO FOOD PLANS

W	Follow recipe as is	**WF**	Follow recipe as is
WS	Not appropriate for the **Rebalance** phase Substitute zucchini for cabbage in **Maintenance** phase Substitute approximately 2 cups Swiss chard for collard in **Rebalance** phase	**WFS**	Not appropriate for the **Rebalance** phase Substitute zucchini for cabbage in **Maintenance** phase

HERB-RUBBED ROASTED DUCK

My nervous system is soothed, and I experience restful sleep after receiving this meal.

*I am thankful for the bird that keeps on giving. This one bird can yield many meals. Duck is a nutrient-dense, easily digestible protein source that is especially high in niacin, phosphorus, riboflavin, iron, zinc, vitamin B6, and thiamine, and contains smaller amounts of vitamin B12, folate, and magnesium. Vitamins B6 and B12 are important in the protection of the cell membrane, red blood cell production, and nervous system function. The herbs used here also yield antibacterial, antimicrobial, antiviral, and immune-supportive benefits. Duck meat is relatively high in fat, so if you are a low-fat **Wildatarian**, opt for only the breast, which is lower in fat than the other parts of the duck.*

— Teri Cochrane

- 4 to 5 pound, bone-in, whole duck
- Freshly squeezed juice from one lemon
- Sea salt
- Coarsely ground black pepper
- ½ pear or apple, cut in quarters
- 1 carrot, cut in half
- One bunch fresh oregano
- One bunch fresh rosemary
- One bunch fresh sage
- 3 tablespoons olive oil

Preheat oven to 425°F. Remove any gizzards, if provided. Rinse duck and pat dry. Place duck on a wire rack in a 10 by 14-inch roasting pan that has been lined with foil. Using a pastry brush, brush on lemon juice. Season bird with salt and pepper. Stuff breast cavity with pear or apple, and carrot. In a small bowl, combine oregano, rosemary, sage, and oil. Mix well to create rub. With a spoon, separate the skin of duck from the breast meat. Apply rub in between skin and breast, then all over the outside of the bird. Bake for 20 minutes. Reduce oven temperature to 350°F; continue baking until meat thermometer registers 135–140°F on the breast. Take duck out of oven. Let stand for 10 to 15 minutes before slicing. Serve with favorite healthful side dishes.

(continued)

APPLICABILITY TO FOOD PLANS

W	Follow recipe as is	WF	Not appropriate for the **Rebalance** phase
WS	Follow recipe as is	WFS	Not appropriate for the **Rebalance** phase

HERB-RUBBED ROASTED DUCK

CONVERTIBLES

This bird can go a long way in converting one meal into several easy convertibles.

BARBECUE DUCK SANDWICHES

- Duck breast, shredded
- Barbecue sauce
- Gluten-free whole grain bun

Shred leftover duck. Toss with your favorite barbeque sauce and then warm. Serve on buns. In minutes, you have barbecue sandwiches!

DUCK, AVOCADO, AND CUCUMBER SANDWICHES

- Duck breast, sliced
- ¼ avocado, sliced
- 4 to 5 cucumber rounds, thinly sliced
- Gluten-free whole grain bread

Layer duck breast slices, avocado, and cucumber rounds on bread.

DUCK AND BEAN ENCHILADA CASSEROLE

- 1½ cups shredded duck
- 2 cans kidney beans, rinsed and drained
- 1 teaspoon cumin
- 1 teaspoon freshly squeezed lime juice
- 1 cup chopped fresh cilantro
- ¼ teaspoon sea salt
- ¼ teaspoon freshly ground black pepper
- 6 gluten-free whole grain tortillas
- 1 cup salsa
- 1 cup shredded Manchego cheese

Preheat oven to 350°F. Combine duck, beans, cumin, lime juice, cilantro, salt, and pepper. Place in a 9 by 12-inch baking dish. Arrange whole grain tortillas in 2 rows of 3 each, with duck mixture in between. Spread salsa on top of tortillas. Top with shredded cheese. Bake for 30 minutes. Broil for 2 minutes or until cheese bubbles. Serve with fresh avocado slices.

Serves 4 to 6.

APPLICABILITY TO FOOD PLANS

W	Follow recipe as is	**WF**	Not appropriate for the **Rebalance** phase
WS	Follow recipe as is	**WFS**	Not appropriate for the **Rebalance** phase

HERBED BUFFALO OR LAMB BURGERS WITH SWEET POTATO "FRIES"

SERVES 6

I feel fit and lean when I consume these burgers and fries.

This is a delicious and nutritious version of the Standard American Diet's burger and fries. You will not miss the grease, fat, or refined carbohydrates that come with the beef burger and white potato fries. Buffalo and bison may be used interchangeably in this recipe. Buffalo has been called the original health food because it is significantly higher in protein while lower in calories, cholesterol, and fat than most other meats. In addition, buffalo is a more easily digestible protein than beef. Buffalo boasts 70 to 90 percent less fat, 50 percent less cholesterol, and 30 percent more protein than beef. Lamb, the alternate choice, is known for its anti-inflammatory fats, which is so important to collagen and skin health. The sweet potatoes are highly alkaline and are rich in fiber, and possess powerful antioxidants.

— Teri Cochrane

HERBED BUFFALO OR LAMB BURGERS

- 1½ pound ground buffalo or ground lamb
- 1 tablespoon dried minced garlic
- 1 teaspoon cracked black pepper
- 1 tablespoon dried oregano
- 1 teaspoon dried parsley
- 1 teaspoon sea salt
- Gluten-free whole grain buns

In a large bowl, combine all ingredients and mix together until well blended. Shape meat into 6 patties. Grill or broil 10 to 15 minutes until cooked to medium, 160°F using a meat thermometer. Serve on buns (optional), or have a naked burger (without a bun).

SWEET POTATO "FRIES"

- 2 medium sweet potatoes, peeled
- 4 teaspoons olive oil, divided
- 1 teaspoon sea salt
- ½ teaspoon cracked black pepper

Preheat oven to 400°F. Lightly coat a 12 by 15-inch baking sheet with 1 teaspoon oil. Cut sweet potatoes lengthwise into strips so they look like standard French fries. Place in a large bowl and toss with remaining oil, salt, and pepper. Arrange potatoes on prepared baking sheet. Bake for 20 to 25 minutes, turning occasionally until golden brown. Serve with burgers.

APPLICABILITY TO FOOD PLANS

W	Follow recipe as is
WS	Eliminate garlic from recipe
WF	Choose buffalo as your wild game meat
WFS	Eliminate garlic from recipe Choose buffalo as your wild game meat

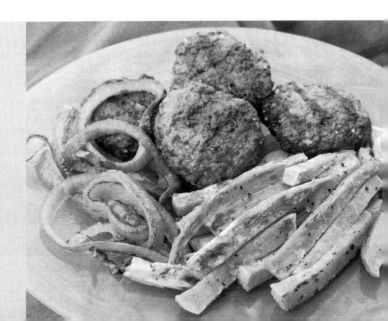

INVITING SMOOTHIES

I joyfully receive abundant health through these colorful phytonutrients.

Smoothies are a palate-friendly way to get kids and adults alike to eat and enjoy different types of fruits and veggies. You can sneak in some less-than-favorite fruits, vegetables, protein sources like flaxseed, and even blood-enrichers like chlorophyll. I am providing two smoothie recipes with a list of "mix-and-match" ingredients that allow you to make your own smoothie combinations. I sometimes freeze the smoothie in Popsicle molds or in champagne glasses for an elegant presentation that can be served as a between-course sorbet when you are entertaining, or even as a light and delicious dessert.

— *Teri Cochrane*

The following two recipes are appropriate for your **Rebalance** phase.

BERRY SMOOTHIE

- One 12-ounce bag frozen mixed berries (strawberries, blueberries, raspberries)
- 1 cup organic unsweetened coconut, almond milk, or cashew milk beverage
- 2 tablespoons monk fruit sugar
- Pinch of sea salt
- 1 tablespoon honey
- ½ avocado
- 1 cup crushed ice

Purée berries in a blender. Add milk, sugar, salt, honey, avocado, and ice; blend until smooth. For thinner consistency, add additional milk. Pour into drinking glasses to serve.

Serves 2 to 4.

For a Frozen Treat: Smoothie mixture can be poured into ice cream shapers and placed into the freezer for 3 to 4 hours.

130

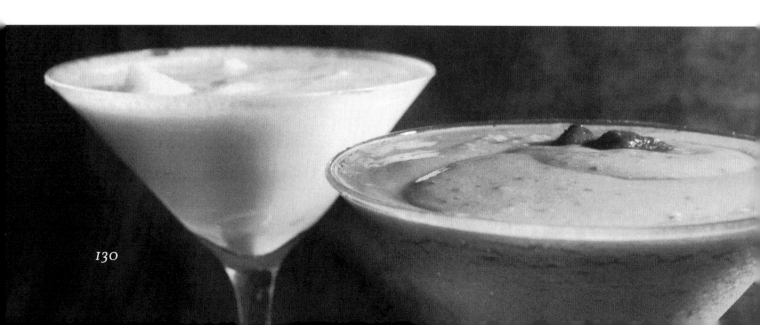

COCONUT AND PAPAYA SMOOTHIE

- 1 cup chopped fresh papaya
- 1 cup canned lite coconut milk
- Pinch of sea salt
- Coconut sugar or monk fruit sugar to desired sweetness
- 1 large cup crushed ice

Purée papaya in a blender. Add coconut milk, salt, sugar, and ice; blend until smooth. For thinner consistency, add additional coconut milk. Pour into drinking glasses to serve.

Serves 2

The mix-and-match-smoothies below should be used during your **Maintenance** phase.

MIX-AND-MATCH SMOOTHIES

These are general guidelines for your mix-and-match smoothies to achieve the proper consistency. Always use 1 cup of liquid in your mix-and-match selection.

- 2 cups fruit (any fresh fruit works well, but best are berries and/or sweet citrus)
- 1 cup greens (spinach, kale, collards, Swiss chard, beet greens, parsley, and/or cilantro)
- 1 cup milk and juices (coconut or almond milk; or carrot, cherry, blueberry, or papaya juice)
- ½ cup nectars (pear, papaya, and/or mango)
- 2 tablespoons seeds (flaxseed, sunflower, or pumpkin)
- 2 tablespoons nut butters (almond, cashew, or sunflower)
- ½ avocado
- Monk fruit or coconut sugar, to taste

Suggested Combinations
- Strawberries, carrot, monk fruit or coconut sugar, avocado, and almond milk
- Applesauce, grape, almond milk, and almond butter
- Peach, pear, papaya, avocado, and sunflower seeds
- Banana, monk fruit or coconut sugar, almond milk, and sunflower butter. *If using banana, only use ½ banana as it may overpower the flavor of the other fruits.*
- Berries, monk fruit or coconut sugar, spinach, and almond milk

APPLICABILITY TO FOOD PLANS

W	Not appropriate for the **Rebalance** phase		**WF**	Not appropriate for the **Rebalance** phase Eliminate nut butters from recipe
WS	Not appropriate for the **Rebalance** phase Eliminate kale and collards from recipe		**WFS**	Not appropriate for the **Rebalance** phase Eliminate kale and collards from recipe Eliminate nut butters from recipe

ITALIAN-STYLE BUFFALO MEAT SAUCE

SERVES 6

I am free from inflammation and strong enough to seize the day.

Oregano and basil are featured in this authentic sauce. Oregano is a known antibacterial and antifungal and has been shown to inhibit the growth of bacteria, including Staphylococcus aureus, which has become resistant to many commonly used antibiotics. Oregano is also great when trying to eliminate yeast from your system. The flavonoids found in basil help protect the all-important DNA. These flavonoids also help to block inflammatory enzymes in the body. Replacing beef with buffalo gives this dish a better flavor, and helps to eliminate the inflammatory response that can occur from consuming beef. Buffalo and bison may be used interchangeably in this recipe. Enjoy this sauce over gluten-free whole grain or brown rice pasta, or even brown basmati rice.

— *Teri Cochrane*

- ¼ chopped onion
- ½ chopped red pepper, ribs and seeds removed
- 5 cloves minced garlic
- ½ teaspoon sea salt
- 1½ pound ground buffalo meat
- ¼ teaspoon cracked black pepper
- 2 tablespoons olive oil
- One 8-ounce can tomato sauce
- One 14-ounce can fire roasted tomatoes (Muir Glen)
- One 6-ounce can tomato paste
- ⅓ cup chopped fresh parsley
- ⅓ cup chopped fresh basil
- ¼ cup chopped fresh oregano
- ¼ cup red wine
- 2 tablespoons filtered water, or more if needed

Heat oil in large saucepan over medium heat. Sauté onion, red pepper, garlic, salt, cracked black pepper, and ground buffalo in oil about 5 to 7 minutes, until meat crumbles and is cooked through. Drain and discard excess liquid. Stir in tomato sauce, tomatoes, tomato paste, parsley, basil, oregano, and red wine. Bring to a low boil, reduce heat, and simmer for approximately 20 to 25 minutes. If sauce is too thick, add water as needed to thin it to the desired consistency. Serve over brown rice or gluten-free whole-grain pasta.

APPLICABILITY TO FOOD PLANS

W	Follow recipe as is	WF	Follow recipe as is
WS	Eliminate garlic from recipe	WFS	Eliminate garlic from recipe

LOW COUNTRY SHRIMP AND CHEESE QUINOA

Substantial and savory proteins safeguard my tissues and joints.

This high-class recipe from the low country is a perfect one-dish meal for easy entertaining. To make this dish an all-protein meal, I have used quinoa instead of traditional corn grits, which offer little other than simple carbohydrates that turn quickly to sugar in our bodies. The texture of the quinoa is a great companion for the cheese. You will feel satiated but not overly full. Shrimp has anti-inflammatory properties, which are beneficial for rheumatoid arthritis and helpful in the prevention of Alzheimer's disease. A word of caution: if you have gout, then shrimp is not your friend; substitute a firm white fish for the shrimp.

— Teri Cochrane

- 4 cups water
- 2 cups quinoa
- ¼ teaspoon sea salt
- ¼ teaspoon cracked black pepper
- 2 tablespoons butter
- 2 cups shredded Manchego cheese
- 1 pound shrimp, peeled and deveined
- 3 cloves garlic, minced
- 1 teaspoon plus one tablespoon olive oil, divided
- 1 teaspoon turmeric
- 1 teaspoon paprika
- ½ cup chopped fresh parsley

In a medium saucepan, bring water to a boil. Add the quinoa, salt, and pepper. Whisk to mix well. Reduce the heat to low. Cover and cook the quinoa until all the water is absorbed, about 10 to 15 minutes. Remove quinoa from heat and stir in the butter and cheese. Keep covered until ready to serve. In a medium bowl, toss shrimp with garlic, 1 teaspoon olive oil, turmeric, and paprika. Heat remaining oil over medium heat in a skillet or pan and sauté shrimp until tender. Cook until shrimp is pink, 2 to 5 minutes. Do not overcook. Add parsley and let wilt. Spoon the quinoa into individual serving bowls. Pour the shrimp mixture over the quinoa.

APPLICABILITY TO FOOD PLANS

W	Follow recipe as is
WS	Eliminate garlic from recipe
WF	Not appropriate for the **Rebalance** phase Reduce the amount of cheese by half in **Maintenance** phase
WFS	Not appropriate for the **Rebalance** phase Eliminate garlic from recipe Reduce the amount of cheese by half in **Maintenance** phase

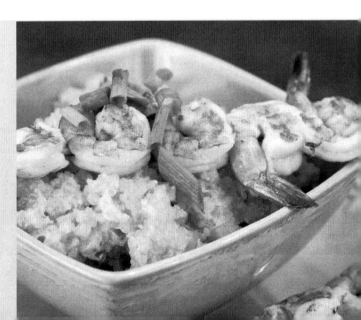

MANGO AND BLACK BEAN SALAD

SERVES 4

I am fortified through nature's sweetness.

This refreshing summertime favorite provides a significant source of iodine, iron, and fiber. Mango, known for its sweetness and beautiful colors, is replete with minerals and antioxidants, especially iodine, iron, and quercetin. Iodine levels in the United States have fallen 50 percent over the last thirty years, and low iodine levels contribute to hypothyroidism. The thyroid gland needs iodine to function properly. The high iron content in mangoes is beneficial to those who are anemic, and the quercetin acts as a natural antihistamine. Mangoes also contain bromelain, a soothing enzyme that helps to digest the beans.

— *Teri Cochrane*

- 1 cup chopped fresh mango
- One 15-ounce can black beans, rinsed and drained
- ½ cup chopped green onion
- ½ chopped red pepper, seeds and ribs removed
- 1 tablespoon freshly squeezed lime juice
- ¼ teaspoon sea salt
- 1 teaspoon cumin
- ¼ teaspoon cracked pepper

Combine all ingredients in a large bowl. Chill for 15 minutes. Serve over field greens or as a side to any wild game or fish main course.

APPLICABILITY TO FOOD PLANS

W	Substitute papaya for mango in **Rebalance** phase	
WS	Eliminate green onion from recipe in **Rebalance** phase Substitute papaya for mango in **Rebalance** phase	

WF	Substitute papaya for mango in **Rebalance** phase	
WFS	Eliminate green onion from recipe in **Rebalance** phase Substitute papaya for mango in **Rebalance** phase	

MEDITERRANEAN-STYLE QUINOA SALAD

These healthful proteins, fats, and carbohydrates give me perfect balance.

High in protein and fiber, this side or main dish is an especially good choice if you are pressed for time. Beautiful in presentation, it takes fewer than 5 minutes to prepare! Best of all, it will make you feel beautiful on the inside because of the nutritional benefits you will be receiving. Quinoa, the salad's main ingredient, is loaded with health benefits. It is a complete protein, and it is high in manganese, magnesium, iron, copper, and phosphorous—all great minerals that are especially helpful to those who experience migraines. The chickpeas are a great source of fiber, which prevents blood sugar levels from rising too rapidly after a meal. Their high molybdenum content may help in detoxifying sulfites, and they are great for those with a sulfur sensitivity. An example of synthetic sulfites are those nasty preservatives found in prepared and packaged foods. The olives, once considered sacred fruits from the Mediterranean region, lend a nice flavor to the quinoa. These little black gems are a good source of the good-for-us fats and vitamin E.

— Teri Cochrane

- 2 cups cooked quinoa
- ½ cup canned chickpeas, rinsed and drained
- ½ cup fresh chopped parsley
- ½ chopped red pepper, seeds and ribs removed
- 1 cup black olives, sliced
- 2 tablespoons olive oil
- 1 tablespoon freshly squeezed lemon juice
- Sea salt
- Cracked pepper
- ½ cup crumbled goat feta cheese

In a large bowl, combine quinoa, chickpeas, parsley, red pepper, black olives, olive oil, and lemon juice. Season with salt and pepper to taste. Top with feta cheese.

APPLICABILITY TO FOOD PLANS

W	Follow recipe as is
WS	Follow recipe as is
WF	Use light/low-fat goat feta
WFS	Use light/low-fat goat feta

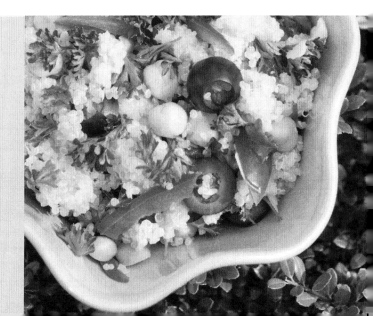

PLUM BOATS WITH BASIL AND GOAT CHEESE

My life force is strengthened through these beneficial antioxidants.

You can make this appetizer or snack in a snap, and everyone will want the recipe. News of this enticing appetizer has spread quickly beyond my client base and into their friends' homes. Most snack food these days is not really food at all, but this one is brimming with good nutrition. Basil boasts antimicrobial properties, and studies coming out of Texas AgriLife Research Center show that plums may have as many or more antioxidants as blueberries. Goat cheese is a great source of calcium, and it is more easily digestible than cow cheese due to its higher pH, shorter-chain fatty acids, and smaller fat molecules.

— Teri Cochrane

- 4 fresh plums, pitted and sliced
- 4 ounces herbed goat cheese
- ½ cup fresh basil leaves, thinly sliced
- 1 teaspoon apple cider vinegar
- 1 teaspoon monk fruit sugar

Place plums on a serving dish. Top plums with goat cheese and basil. Combine vinegar and sugar and stir until sugar is dissolved. Drizzle vinegar/sugar combination over cheese.

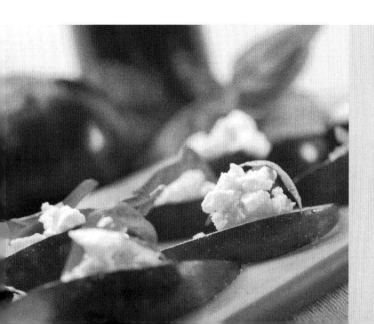

APPLICABILITY TO FOOD PLANS

W	Substitute kiwi for plums in **Rebalance** phase
WS	Substitute kiwi for plums in **Rebalance** phase
WF	Substitute kiwi for plums in **Rebalance** phase Substitute Manchego for goat cheese in **Rebalance** phase
WFS	Substitute kiwi for plums in **Rebalance** phase Substitute Manchego for goat cheese in **Rebalance** phase

PROTEIN RICH RASPBERRY BROWNIES

Rich flavors sweetly satisfy me.

This is not my recipe, but instead, an adaptation from one given to me by a friend. These brownies are so healthful that you will be tempted to eat them for breakfast, but save them for your afternoon or evening treat. This flourless brownie uses chickpeas as its base. Chickpeas give this dessert ample fiber (nearly 10 grams per serving), and a healthful helping of protein. Their high fiber content helps to manage blood sugar levels, which is especially hard to do when you eat sweet treats. Using monk fruit sugar also helps to lower the glycemic index of this fudgy and rich brownie.

— Teri Cochrane

- Coconut oil for greasing pan
- One 14-ounce can chickpeas, rinsed and drained
- 4 medium eggs, at room temperature
- ¼ teaspoon salt
- 1 teaspoon baking powder
- One 12-ounce package semisweet or dark chocolate chips
- ¼ cup monk fruit sugar
- ⅓ cup avocado or grapeseed oil
- One 12-ounce bag frozen raspberries, thawed and drained

Preheat oven to 350 degrees F. Oil an 8 by 8-inch square baking pan. Place chickpeas in a food processor, and pulse until pureed. In a large mixing bowl, beat 4 eggs with an electric mixer. Mix in salt, baking powder, and chickpeas; set aside. Melt chocolate chips in a double boiler over medium-low heat. Remove from heat and let cool to room temperature. Whisk chocolate into egg mixture until well blended. Slowly add monk fruit sugar, to taste, for sweetness. Add oil and mix well, then fold in raspberries. Place batter in prepared pan. Bake for 35 to 40 minutes, or until a toothpick inserted into the center comes out clean.

Note: If you do not have a double boiler, place chips in a metal bowl (or smaller pan) over a pan of boiling water. Do not let the water touch the bottom of the bowl. Stir chips until they have melted.

APPLICABILITY TO FOOD PLANS

W	Not appropriate for the **Rebalance** phase
WS	Not appropriate for the **Rebalance** phase
WF	Not appropriate for the **Rebalance** phase
WFS	Not appropriate for the **Rebalance** phase

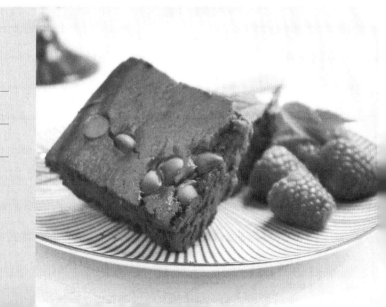

PUMPKIN BUCKWHEAT CREPES

I am satiated by healthful sweets.

This high-protein dessert or breakfast option will have everyone wanting more. The pumpkin provides the moisture needed, so no oil is used. Buckwheat is a near complete protein, containing eight of the nine essential amino acids, and is a gluten-free seed grain. Pairing these crepes with blueberries provides a burst of fresh flavor, and their color complements the slightly purple color of the crepes.

— *Teri Cochrane*

- 3 eggs
- ½ teaspoon vanilla extract
- 4 tablespoons pumpkin puree
- 1 cup pasture fed organic milk (use a milk substitute, if necessary)
- 1 cup buckwheat flour, sifted
- ½ teaspoon salt
- ⅓ cup pure cane organic sugar
- ¼ cup chopped basil
- 1 cup blueberries, divided
- 2 tablespoons honey
- ¼ teaspoon lemon juice
- 1 cup whipped cream (optional)

Heat griddle to 350°F. Whisk eggs. Add vanilla, pumpkin, and milk. Mix well and set aside. Combine flour, salt, and sugar. Add dry ingredients and basil (if using) to the liquid mixture. With a dry ¼-cup measuring cup, pour batter onto griddle. Spread batter evenly into large, thin, oval-shaped crepes, leaving enough room on griddle between crepes to allow them to be flipped. Cook until golden brown. Flip crepes. Once bottoms are golden brown, remove crepes from griddle, and keep warm. Repeat process until all batter has been used. In a medium bowl, toss blueberries with honey and lemon juice. Place one tablespoon blueberry mixture on each crepe. Top with whipped cream (optional).

APPLICABILITY TO FOOD PLANS

W	Not appropriate for the **Rebalance** phase	**WF**	Not appropriate for the **Rebalance** phase
WS	Not appropriate for the **Rebalance** phase	**WFS**	Not appropriate for the **Rebalance** phase

QUINOA WITH CINNAMON, APPLES, AND WALNUTS

I begin each day fully nourished, and I am complete.

Apples and walnuts help to add fiber and flavor to a high protein breakfast option. This also can be served as a simple dessert or an afternoon snack. Walnuts are an especially high source of omega-3 fatty acids; just ¼ cup nearly meets your daily allowance for this beneficial fat. Apples are high in the bioflavonoids quercetin, catechin, and phloridzin; they support lung health and protect against osteoporosis and even breast cancer. I have purposely left the skin on the apples because that is where many of the health benefits reside. I strongly encourage purchasing organic varieties to minimize exposure to harmful pesticides and waxes.

— *Teri Cochrane*

- 1 cup dry quinoa
- 2 cups water
- Pinch of sea salt
- 1 tablespoon butter
- 3 Gala or Fuji apples, washed, unpeeled, and sliced
- 1 teaspoon ground cinnamon
- ½ cup chopped walnuts
- 2 teaspoons honey

Thoroughly rinse and drain quinoa in a mesh colander. Place first 3 ingredients in a 3-quart pot. Cover and bring to a boil. Lower heat to simmer, and cook about 15 minutes or until quinoa has expanded. Let butter melt in a large cast iron skillet over medium heat. Add apples and cinnamon; stir to combine. Cook apples until just tender, about 5 minutes. Place quinoa in individual serving bowls, and top with warm apple mixture, walnuts, and one teaspoon honey. Serve with coconut, brown rice, or almond milk.

CONVERTIBLE

QUINOA WITH BERRIES, PEACHES, AND PUMPKIN SEEDS

Replace apples with fresh berries, fresh peach slices, and pumpkin seeds.

APPLICABILITY TO FOOD PLANS

W	Not appropriate for the **Rebalance** phase
WS	Not appropriate for the **Rebalance** phase
WF	Not appropriate for the **Rebalance** phase
WFS	Not appropriate for the **Rebalance** phase

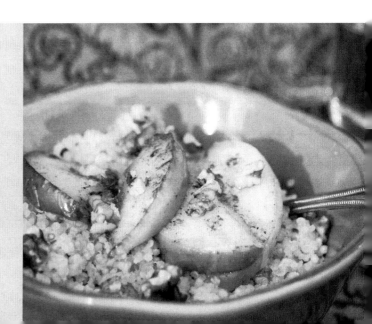

RED BEANS AND RICE

Fiber supports me every day in every way.

This dish brings together two cultures and cuisines: brown basmati rice from India and red beans from the Deep South of the United States. Basmati rice has a nutty flavor, which cools the hot spices used for the beans. Red beans are the king of beans in terms of fiber. One cup of cooked red beans contains almost 20 grams of fiber, which helps lead the way toward a total recommended daily minimum of 30 grams. New research finds that beans also top the list in terms of antioxidants. USDA lists red beans as number one in their top 20 best sources of antioxidants, as measured by the total antioxidant content per serving. Using canned beans in this recipe makes this meal not only really easy to make, but also better for anyone whose digestive system is bothered by beans. The natural sugar in beans is what contributes to digestive discomfort. With canned beans, some of sugar migrates from the beans to the liquid in which they've been cooked. Rinsing and draining the canned beans can help lower their gas-causing effects. Together, the rice and beans create a complete protein—a must especially for those who do not consume animal proteins.

— Teri Cochrane

- 1½ cups basmati brown rice
- 1 teaspoon sea salt, divided
- 3 cups filtered water
- ½ tablespoon olive oil
- 3 cloves garlic, minced
- ¼ medium yellow onion, chopped
- Pinch of ground black pepper
- Two 15-ounce cans of red beans, any variety
- One 14-ounce can diced tomatoes, undrained
- 1 teaspoon chili powder
- 1 teaspoon paprika
- 2 teaspoons Tabasco® sauce
- 1 tablespoon cumin

In a medium saucepan, add rice, ½ teaspoon salt, and water. Bring to a boil. Reduce to a simmer, cover, and cook on low heat for approximately 50 minutes. Over medium heat in a medium skillet, heat olive oil and sauté garlic, onion, and pepper until tender, about 5 minutes. Add beans, tomatoes, ½ teaspoon salt, chili powder, paprika, Tabasco, and cumin. Cook on medium heat for approximately 15 minutes, until sauce thickens slightly. Spoon rice onto individual plates and top with beans.

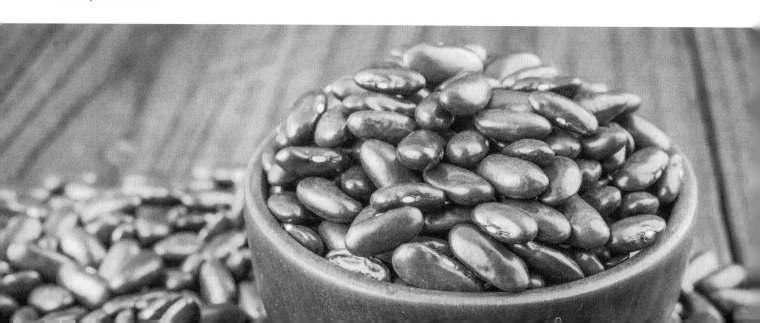

CONVERTIBLE

RED BEAN DIP

- 1 cup cooked beans
- ¼ teaspoon freshly squeezed lime juice
- ¼ teaspoon sea salt
- ½ chunky salsa (any brand)
- ¼ cup of chopped fresh cilantro

Mix prepared beans, lime juice, sea salt; and salsa. Top with cilantro. You can either puree the dip or serve as is.

Serves 4.

APPLICABILITY TO FOOD PLANS

W	Follow recipe as is	WF	Follow recipe as is
WS	Eliminate garlic from recipe	WFS	Eliminate garlic from recipe

SAVORY SLOPPY JOES GO WILD

SERVES 4 TO 6

Caribbean spices, healthy lipids, and proteins give me strength and vigor.

This version of Sloppy Joes takes away all the unhealthy fats, proteins, and preservatives found in traditional versions. And they are so easy to make!

— *Teri Cochrane*

- ½ onion, minced
- 2 cloves garlic
- ½ green pepper, seeds and ribs removed, chopped
- 1 teaspoon dried oregano
- ½ teaspoon sea salt
- 2 pounds ground buffalo (or bison) or ground elk or a combination of the two
- One 14-ounce can tomato sauce
- One 16-ounce jar Bone Suckin' Sauce®

In a large skillet over medium heat, sauté onions, garlic, pepper, oregano, sea salt, and buffalo and/or elk for about 10 minutes, until cooked through and crumbly. Add tomato and barbecue sauces. Cook, stirring occasionally, until sauces are absorbed.

APPLICABILITY TO FOOD PLANS

W	Follow recipe as is	WF	Follow recipe as is
WS	Eliminate garlic from recipe	WFS	Eliminate garlic from recipe

SAVORY SPICED PECANS AND ALMONDS

MAKES 8 ONE-HALF
CUP SERVINGS

I receive foods that support good health and well-being.

Incorporating nuts into our daily fare is important for providing healthful proteins, beneficial oils, and vitamins. Almonds are my favorite type of nut. I consume them multiple times throughout the day in small doses. Almonds are rich in vitamin E, and both almonds and pecans supply magnesium, potassium, and calcium. Both types of nuts have been shown to lower LDL cholesterol and stabilize blood sugar levels. New studies are proving that the essential fatty acids in these types of nuts may help promote weight loss with moderate daily consumption, and they can help lower the incidence of stroke and heart disease.

— Teri Cochrane

- 2 cups raw whole pecans
- 2 cups raw whole almonds
- 6 cups filtered water
- ⅓ cup turbinado sugar
- 1 teaspoon cayenne pepper
- 1 teaspoon salt
- Coconut oil for greasing cookie sheet

Preheat oven to 350°F. Lightly grease two stainless steel jelly-roll pans. Place almonds and pecans in a medium saucepan. Cover with water. Bring to boil, remove from heat, and drain. In a separate bowl, add sugar, pepper, and salt. Mix in nuts to fully coat them with the sugar mixture. Spread nuts evenly on prepared cookie sheets. Bake for approximately 15 to 20 minutes, until sugar is caramelized and nuts are golden brown, turning occasionally so that they do not burn. Remove from heat. Immediately place nuts on waxed or parchment paper, and let cool until they are dry. Serve as a dessert with cheese or top salad greens with them.

APPLICABILITY TO FOOD PLANS

W	Not appropriate for the **Rebalance** phase
WS	Not appropriate for the **Rebalance** phase
WF	Not appropriate for the **Rebalance** phase
WFS	Not appropriate for the **Rebalance** phase

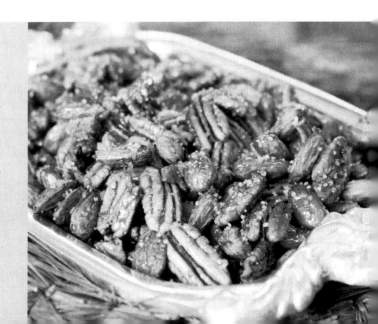

TEA BLENDS AND FLAVORED WATERS

I am soothed by and replenished with these healthful libations.

Warm or cold beverages comfort us and quench our thirst. These fresh offerings are ideal alternatives to sodas or commercial teas that are riddled with high fructose syrup, artificial dyes, and preservatives. The natural sweetness of fruits, herbs, and honey can flavor water in a way that is very satisfying and enjoyable. Mint is a coolant to our systems; pineapple and cinnamon offer digestive aids; and chamomile and black cherry are soothing anti-inflammatory agents. You will love the flavors that can be infused into simple water.

— Teri Cochrane

CINNAMON COCONUT LATTE

- 4 cups water
- 4 cinnamon sticks
- 1 cup unsweetened coconut milk beverage, warmed

In a medium sauce pot, bring water to a boil. Remove from stove and add cinnamon sticks. Cover and let steep for 10 minutes. Remove cinnamon sticks and place one in each of four mugs. Pour 1 cup cinnamon tea and add ¼ cup coconut milk into each mug, and serve.

Serves 4

APPLICABILITY TO FOOD PLANS

W, WS, WF, WFS	Follow recipe as is

PINEAPPLE WATER

- 1 quart sparkling water
- 2 cups fresh pineapple chunks

Place water and pineapple in a glass pitcher. Cover and refrigerate for at least 4 hours. Serve.

Serves 4

APPLICABILITY TO FOOD PLANS

W, WS, WF, WFS	Substitute 2 cups of fresh watermelon and ½ cup of papaya chunks for pineapple in recipe during the **Rebalance** phase

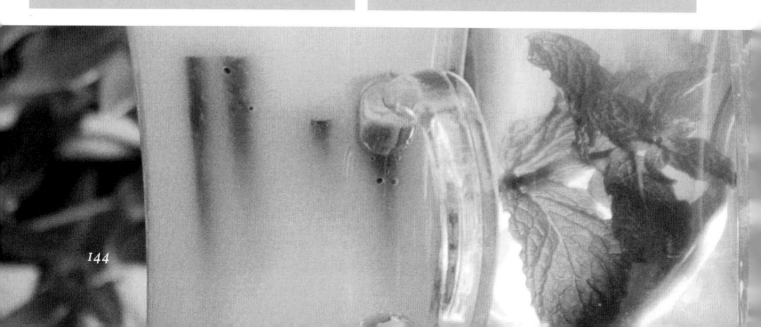

MINT, CHAMOMILE, HONEY, AND GREEN TEA

- 1 quart water
- 1 green tea bag
- 1 chamomile tea bag
- ½ cup fresh mint leaves
- ¼ cup honey

Place water in a teapot or saucepan and bring to a boil. Remove from heat. Add tea bags, mint, and honey. Cover and let steep for 5 to 10 minutes. Serve warm or pour over ice for an iced tea treat.

Serves 4

APPLICABILITY TO FOOD PLANS

W, WS, WF, WFS	Substitute monk fruit sugar for honey in **Rebalance** phase Follow recipe as is in **Maintenance** phase

ARONIA POMATINI

- 1 cup aronia or black cherry juice
- ½ cup papaya nectar
- 1 cup pomegranate juice
- 1 teaspoon freshly squeezed lime juice
- ½ cup sparkling water

Pour all ingredients into a glass pitcher. Add 1 cup of ice. Stir or shake as you would when making a martini. Using a mesh colander, strain drink into martini glasses. Serve immediately.

Serves 4

APPLICABILITY TO FOOD PLANS

W, WS, WF, WFS	Not appropriate for the **Rebalance** phase Use recipe as is for the **Maintenance** phase

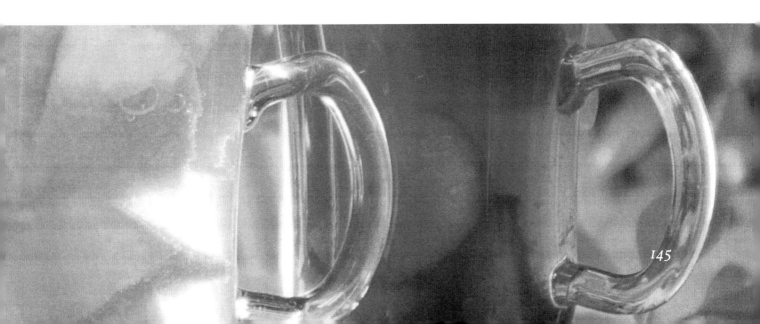

THAI BASIL, COCONUT, AND CURRY SQUASH SOUP

SERVES 6

My body is protected at the cellular level by this delicious and elegant soup.

This is a two-meals-in-one recipe and one of my convertible meals. First, use wild boar to make the broth for the soup. Then, use the meat for sandwiches or shred it to make **Wild Boar Carnitas.** Winter squash, such as butternut, is abundant in beta-carotene, which has been shown to have very powerful antioxidant and anti-inflammatory properties. Studies also show that regular intake of beta-carotene can help reduce the risk of colon cancer, possibly by protecting colon cells from the effects of cancer-causing chemicals. Coconut milk has antiviral and anti-carcinogenic properties. The flavonoids in basil are antimicrobial, which fight disease and help protect us at the cellular level. What a triple threat to cancer cells!

— *Teri Cochrane*

- 8 cups filtered water
- ½ pound wild boar rump (for broth only)
- 1 medium onion, cut into thick slices
- 1 medium butternut squash, peeled and cubed with seeds removed
- 1 teaspoon sea salt, or more to taste
- One 14-ounce can organic coconut milk
- ½ teaspoon curry powder
- ½ teaspoon ground ginger
- Pinch of turbinado sugar
- ½ cup fresh basil leaves (stacked, rolled, and cut crosswise and then measured)

In a large pot over high heat, place water, wild boar, onion, squash, and salt; bring to a boil. Reduce heat to medium, and simmer for approximately 35 minutes or until wild boar is cooked thoroughly. Remove wild boar from pot, set aside. Stir in coconut milk, curry, ginger, and sugar. Mix well to combine. With a hand immersion blender or food processor, purée soup. Add additional salt if desired. Spoon puréed soup into individual bowls. Garnish with basil leaves, allow leaves to wilt, and serve.

Note: To make this a purely vegetarian soup, omit the wild boar.

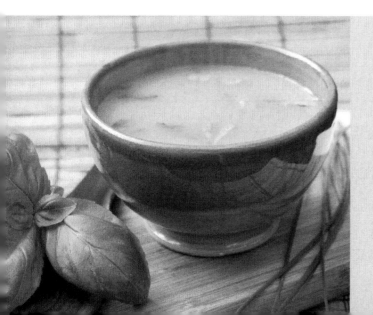

APPLICABILITY TO FOOD PLANS

W	Follow recipe as is
WS	Follow recipe as is
WF	Not appropriate for the **Rebalance** phase
WFS	Not appropriate for the **Rebalance** phase

TOMATO, BASIL, AND GOAT CHEESE FRITTATA

I am free-spirited enough to make the best food choices for my body.

I think this is one of the easiest egg dishes to prepare. It can be served any time of day; just dress it up or down. The best thing is that you can play around with different ingredients to make a different version every time. My rules are that the ingredients must be fresh and good for you. Eggs are the closest protein to mother's milk, as they have a biological quality greater than any other natural food. This means that all of its amino acids are used efficiently by the body. Eggs deliver liver protective benefits. The egg yolks, however, are a very rich source of sulfur, so avoid them if you are sulfur sensitive. A few other frittata versions have been provided, but let the fresh herbs and vegetables in your refrigerator guide you to what will be in your next frittata.

— Teri Cochrane

- 1 tablespoon olive oil
- ½ medium onion, chopped
- 12 medium organic eggs
- ¼ teaspoon sea salt
- ¼ teaspoon cracked black pepper
- ⅔ cup chopped fresh basil,
- 2 cups grape tomatoes sliced in half
- ½ cup Manchego cheese

In a 12-inch cast iron skillet, heat olive oil and sauté onions over medium heat. Crack eggs and place in a large mixing bowl. Add salt and pepper. Whisk eggs until well-mixed. Pour egg mixture into skillet; lift edges of egg mixture so the undercooked part can run onto the skillet. Keep lifting edges of the egg mixture so it becomes uniformly cooked, about 5 minutes. Add basil, and continue to lift edges of egg mixture. When the mixture is cooked on the bottom and partially set, place tomatoes evenly on top of egg mixture. Top with cheese, spreading cheese evenly. Remove from stove and place skillet under broiler for 2 to 3 minutes, until cheese bubbles. Remove from oven, and let skillet cool. Cut frittata into wedges. Serve with salad or avocado and salsa.

(continued)

APPLICABILITY TO FOOD PLANS

W	Follow recipe as is
WS	Not appropriate for the **Rebalance** phase
WF	Not appropriate for the **Rebalance** phase
WFS	Not appropriate for the **Rebalance** phase

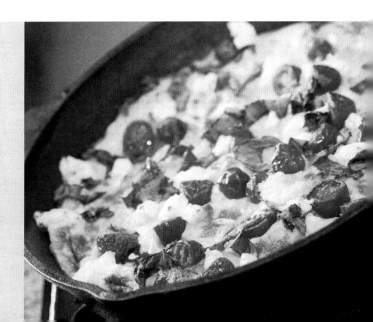

TOMATO, BASIL, AND GOAT CHEESE FRITTATA

(continued)

CONVERTIBLES

Here are some variations for this recipe:

GREEN FRITTATA

- 1 cup fresh broccoli florets
- ½ chopped green pepper (ribs and seeds removed)
- 1 cup raw spinach
- ½ cup chopped fresh parsley

Add these ingredients to the basic egg mixture.

ASPARAGUS FETA FRITTATA

- 1 cup fresh asparagus tips
- ½ cup feta cheese

Add these ingredients to the basic egg mixture.

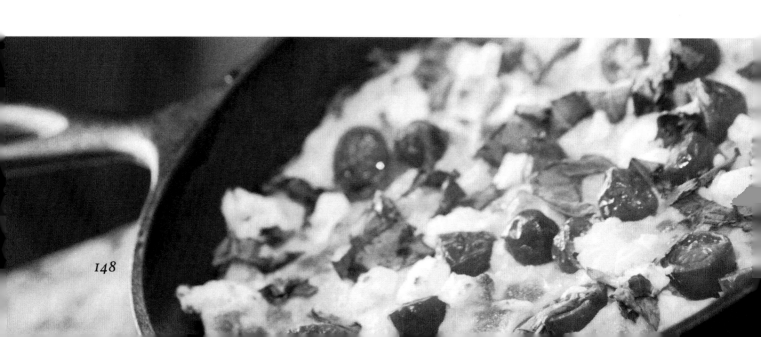

WILD BLUEBERRY, QUINOA, AND OAT BARS

SERVES 8 TO 10

Perfect protein and fiber deliciously satisfy my taste buds and my body; I am grateful.

The oat and quinoa combination will provide a high-protein, high-fiber, yummy alternative to the standard muffins loaded with refined flours, preservatives, and food dyes. I love this in the morning, but it is also one of my favorite afternoon snacks when I need something a little sweet. These bars will help you get through your afternoon slump and manage your sugar cravings while keeping your blood sugar levels stable. The quinoa also provides a complete protein to keep you satiated. Combining the flours with wild blueberries imparts a wonderful antioxidant benefit. Dried blueberries can carry up to four times the level of antioxidants of their fresh counterparts.

— *Teri Cochrane*

- Coconut oil for greasing pan
- 2 cups oat flour
- 2 cups quinoa flour
- 2 tablespoons aluminum-free baking powder
- ½ teaspoon sea salt
- ½ teaspoon cinnamon
- ⅔ cup honey
- 2 cups organic almond milk
- 1 cup unsweetened applesauce
- 1 teaspoon vanilla extract
- 2 large eggs, beaten
- 1½ to 2 cups dried blueberries
- 1 cup chopped almonds

Preheat oven to 350°F. Lightly oil an 11 by 7 by 1 ½-inch baking dish. In a large bowl, stir together the flours, baking powder, salt, and cinnamon. Add honey, milk, applesauce, vanilla, and eggs. Fold in blueberries. Pour into prepared pan and bake for approximately 15 minutes. Open oven and top batter with chopped almonds. Bake for an additional 20 to 25 minutes or until toothpick comes out clean. Cut into squares and serve warm with nut butter or honey.

APPLICABILITY TO FOOD PLANS

W	Not appropriate for the **Rebalance** phase
WS	Not appropriate for the **Rebalance** phase
WF	Not appropriate for the **Rebalance** phase
WFS	Not appropriate for the **Rebalance** phase

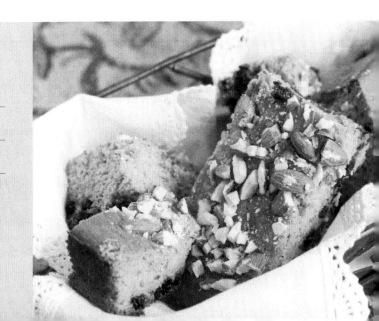

WILD BOAR CARNITAS

This quick and easy meal lets me make "fast food" in my own home.

If you plan ahead, this is an awesome, quick, on-the-go meal. You will be able to wrap and roll this meal in less than 5 minutes, if your wild boar is already cooked. All you need to do is shred the meat and place the ingredients in the pan. Wild boar replaces traditional pork, which has now been linked to a host of gastrointestinal conditions because of the potential pathogens it carries.

— Teri Cochrane

- 8 cups filtered water
- ½ onion, cut into quarters
- 1 stalk celery, cut into chunks
- 1 teaspoon sea salt
- 1 teaspoon dried oregano
- 1 pound wild boar rump

Seasoning Mixture:

- 1 onion sliced thinly
- ½ teaspoon salt
- 1 teaspoon ground cumin
- ½ teaspoon crumbled dried oregano
- Juice from one lime
- 1 tablespoon olive oil

In a stock pot over high heat, bring water, onion, celery, salt, oregano, and wild boar to a boil. Reduce heat to medium-low and simmer uncovered for approximately 35 minutes or until meat is cooked through. Remove wild boar and shred (keep stock for soup; see Convertibles recipe below). Transfer shredded wild boar to a medium bowl. Add seasoning mixture ingredients, except for olive oil, and toss together. Add olive oil to a non-stick skillet and toss in wild boar mixture. Stir-fry over high heat for 3 to 5 minutes. Serve with rice, beans, and gluten-free whole grain tortillas.

CONVERTIBLE

WILD BOAR STOCK VEGETABLE SOUP

- 4 cups stock
- 1 bag frozen vegetables
- One 14.5-ounce can of tomatoes

Use stock to make a quick and easy soup with organic veggies and canned tomatoes.

APPLICABILITY TO FOOD PLANS

W	Follow recipe as is	**WF**	Follow recipe as is
WS	Eliminate celery from recipe	**WFS**	Eliminate celery from recipe

WILD GAME CHILI

My heart is strengthened, and I am filled with gratitude for these flavorful spices.

This recipe is a favorite of my clients. Even beginners in the kitchen find it easy to prepare. The spices work together to give this meal its great flavor. But the spices used are more than just tasty. They possess potent antimicrobial and anti-inflammatory properties that provide significant protection against several chronic health conditions, including heart disease and tumor formation.

— Teri Cochrane

- 1 tablespoon olive oil
- 2 pounds ground bison or buffalo, elk, or venison
- ½ cup chopped onion
- ½ cup chopped red pepper
- 3 cloves garlic, minced
- ½ cup water
- 1 teaspoon chili powder (or more to taste)
- 1 tablespoon ground cumin
- ¼ teaspoon nutmeg
- ¼ teaspoon cinnamon
- ¼ teaspoon paprika
- 1 teaspoon turbinado or pure cane sugar
- ½ teaspoon sea salt, or more to taste
- ¼ teaspoon cracked black pepper
- One 16-ounce can pinto beans, drained
- One 16-ounce can chickpeas, drained
- Two 14-ounce cans fire roasted diced tomatoes
- One 8-ounce can tomato sauce
- One 6-ounce can tomato paste
- 1 cup fresh chopped cilantro

In a large Dutch oven, add olive oil, ground meat, onion, red pepper, and garlic. Cook over medium-high heat until meat is browned, stirring until meat crumbles. Add remaining ingredients except cilantro, stirring until well combined. Bring to a boil, reduce heat, and simmer for approximately 20 minutes, stirring occasionally. Spoon into bowls; top with fresh cilantro.

APPLICABILITY TO FOOD PLANS

W	Follow recipe as is		**WF**	Follow recipe as is
WS	Eliminate garlic from recipe		**WFS**	Eliminate garlic from recipe

WILD GAME MEATBALLS

SERVES 6

I am grounded and energized by nourishing protein and energy that allows me to thrive.

These are a fantastic anytime dinner because the recipe can be doubled and tripled, and the leftovers keep well as an easy snack or add-on for lunches or other busy weeknight dinners. The amino acids from the wild game are more bio-available to you then those from conventionally raised meats, which can come loaded with toxins, antibiotics, and hormones. Thank you to Lauren Rice for this delicious recipe.

— Teri Cochrane

- 1 pound of ground elk, bison or buffalo, lamb, or antelope
- 2 to 6 cloves of garlic, to taste
- ¼ cup raw onion
- 4 tablespoons fresh rosemary or dried Herbs de Provence mix or an Italian herb blend
- 1½ teaspoons salt
- ½ teaspoon pepper
- ½ tablespoon butter or healthy oil such as olive, coconut, avocado, or sunflower for browning

Preheat oven to 400°F. Incorporate all ingredients and form into 2-inch balls (for an even interior while browning). Place the balls in large cast-iron or stainless steel skillet, and fry in butter or a healthy oil alternative. Brown and flip. Finish in 400°F oven for 12 to 20 minutes or until cooked to preferred doneness.

Note: Elk, bison, and buffalo are lean, and they may require one egg and 1 cup of a flour for desired consistency, though I have made them without this with tasty results! Grind some baked chickpea snacks, available at most natural grocers, to make excellent breadcrumbs! Nut flours are generally too wet for this task and better reserved for baked goods that require a softer consistency. If using lamb, usually no other binders are necessary due to the slightly higher fat content.

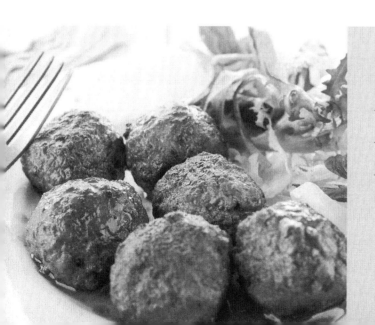

APPLICABILITY TO FOOD PLANS

W	Follow recipe as is
WS	Eliminate garlic in **Rebalance** phase
WF	Do not use lamb in **Rebalance** phase
WFS	Eliminate garlic in **Rebalance** phase Do not use lamb in **Rebalance** phase

WILD GAME MEATLOAF

SERVES 6 TO 8

Smoky and sweet flavors bring forth soothing memories.

This version of meatloaf will leave you completely satisfied, yet not overly full like traditional meatloaf might. Using rolled oats adds fiber and replaces the white starch that comes from nutrient-poor bread crumbs. The sweet flavor of the dried fruit, in combination with the herbs, will remind you of Thanksgiving.

— Teri Cochrane

- Olive oil for coating pan
- 2 pounds ground bison or buffalo, lamb, elk, or wild boar
- ½ medium onion, chopped
- ⅓ cup chopped fresh parsley
- 1 teaspoon dried oregano
- ½ teaspoon dried sage
- ⅓ cup rolled oats
- ⅓ cup monk fruit sugar
- ½ cup dried sulfite-free cherries
- Egg white from one large egg
- 6 ounces of tomato sauce
- 1 cup organic ketchup

Preheat oven to 350°F. Line bottom of broiler pan with aluminum foil and lightly coat slotted broiler tray surface with oil to keep meatloaf from sticking. In a large bowl, place all ingredients except ketchup. Mix together until well blended. Form meat mixture into loaf on top of broiler tray. Spread ketchup over top and sides of loaf. Bake in oven for 1 hour and 10 minutes or until meat thermometer registers 170°F. Remove from oven; let stand for 5 to 10 minutes.

CONVERTIBLE

WILD BURGERS

Don't feel like turning on the oven? Then shape the meat mixture into patties and grill them as burgers for a warm-weather treat!

Turn grill to medium-high heat. Omit ketchup from ingredients. Shape into 8 patties and grill for 10 minutes or until cooked to 170°F using a meat thermometer.

APPLICABILITY TO FOOD PLANS

W	Substitute quinoa flakes for oats in **Rebalance** phase Eliminate cherries from recipe in **Rebalance** phase	**WF**	Substitute quinoa flakes for oats in **Rebalance** phase Eliminate cherries from recipe in **Rebalance** phase Do not choose lamb as your wild meat
WS	Substitute quinoa flakes for oats in **Rebalance** phase Eliminate cherries from recipe in **Rebalance** phase	**WFS**	Substitute quinoa flakes for oats in **Rebalance** phase Eliminate cherries from recipe in **Rebalance** phase Do not choose lamb as your wild meat

WILD SALMON IN PARCHMENT PAPER

SERVES 4

My cell membranes benefit from the richness of these beneficial omega-3s.

This dish is fabulously elegant yet deceptively simple. Your friends and family will think it took you all day to make. Wild-caught salmon is a great protein source, rich in omega-3 and selenium, both of which are protective to the cell membrane. Omega-3 fatty acids are a natural anti-inflammatory and help maintain hormone balance. This fish is also rich in vitamins B6 and B12, both of which are needed for proper production of DNA. Pair this recipe with wild rice or roasted root vegetables to get a high source of vitamins A and E. The antioxidant properties of selenium are increased when paired with these vitamins.

— *Teri Cochrane*

- 4 wild-caught salmon fillets
- 4 sheets parchment paper, each approximately 12 square inches
- 1 tablespoon dried minced garlic, or 3 cloves garlic, minced
- 1 tablespoon dried basil
- 1 tablespoon dried oregano
- 3 tablespoons olive oil, divided
- Freshly squeezed juice from ½ lemon
- Dash of sea salt
- ½ teaspoon fresh cracked black pepper

Preheat oven to 425°F. Place each fillet in the middle of a piece of parchment paper. In a small bowl, mix together garlic (optional), basil, oregano, and 2 tablespoons of olive oil to create herb mixture. Divide the herb mixture into 4 equal parts. Drizzle each fillet with remaining olive oil and the lemon juice. Place herb mixture on fish; sprinkle salt and pepper on top. Fold each piece of parchment paper over the fish fillet, folding and crimping edges tightly to seal and enclose the fish. Place packets on cookie sheet. Bake for 15 to 17 minutes. Open one packet to ensure fish is done and flakes easily. Place packets on individual serving dishes. Serve with brown or wild rice, or quinoa.

APPLICABILITY TO FOOD PLANS

W	Follow recipe as is		**WF**	Substitute halibut, mahi, or snapper for salmon in **Rebalance** phase
WS	Eliminate garlic from recipe		**WFS**	Eliminate garlic from recipe Substitute halibut, mahi, or snapper for salmon in **Rebalance** phase

BIBLIOGRAPHY

Abu, A. and Basal, M. A. "Healing Potential of *Rosmarinus Officinalis* L. on Full-Thickness Excision Cutaneous Wounds in Alloxan-Induced-Diabetic BALB/c Mice." *Journal of Ethnopharmacology* 131, no. 2 (2010): 443–50.

Agarwal, A. K., Garg, R., Ritch, A., and Sarkar, P. "Postural Orthostatic Tachycardia Syndrome." *Postgraduate Medical Journal* 83, no. 981 (2007): 478–480.

Ahmad, Z. "The Uses and Properties of Almond Oil." *Complementary Therapies in Clinical Practice* 16, no. 1 (February 2010): 10–20.

Akgül, A. and Kivanc, M. "Inhibitory Effects of Selected Turkish Spices and Oregano Components on Some Foodborne Fungi." *International Journal of Food Microbiology* 6, no. 3 (1988): 263–268.

Alexandrescu, A. T. "Amyloid Accomplices and Enforcers." *Protein Science* 14, no. 1 (2005): 1–12, https://doi.org/10.1110/ps.04887005.

American Heart Association. "Whole Grain, Bran Intake Associated with Lower Risk of Death in Diabetic Women." Last modified May 10, 2010. http://www.newsroom.heart.org/index.php?s=43&item=1028.

Andersson, K. E., Svedberg, K. A., Lindholm, M. W., Oste, R., and Hellstrand, P. "Oats (*Avena Sativa*) Reduce Atherogenesis in LDL-Receptor-Deficient Mice." *Atherosclerosis*, 212, no. 1 (Sep 30): 93–99.

Antonious, G. F., Bomford, M., and Vincelli, P. "Screening Brassica Species for Glucosinolate Content." *Journal of Environmental Science and Health*. Part B 44, no. 3 (March 2009): 311–316, PMID: 19280485.

Aparicio, A., Andres, P., Perea, J. M., Lopez-Sobaler, A. M., and Ortega, R. M. "Influence of the Consumption of Fruits and Vegetables on the Nutritional Status of a Group of

Institutionalized Elderly Persons in the Madrid Region." *The Journal of Nutrition, Health, and Aging* 14, no. 8 (2010): 615–620, PMID: 20922336.

Aprikian, O., Duclos, V., Guyot, S., Besson, C., Manach, C., Bernalier, A., Morand, C., Remesy, C. and Demigne, C. "Apple Pectin and a Polyphenol-Rich Apple Concentrate Are More Effective Together than Separately on Cecal Fermentations and Plasma Lipids in Rats." *The Journal of Nutrition* 133, no. 6 (June 2003): 1860–1865.

Aran, A., Lin, L., Finn, L. A., Weiner, K., Peppard, P., Young, T., and Mignot, E. "Post-streptococcal Antibodies Are Associated with Metabolic Syndrome in a Population-Based Cohort." *PLoS ONE* 6, no. 9 (2011): e25017.

Aran, A., Weiner, K., Lin, L., Finn, L. A., Greco, M. A., Peppard, P., Young, T., Ofran, Y., and Mignot, E. "Post-streptococcal Auto-antibodies Inhibit Protein Disulfide Isomerase and Are Associated with Insulin Resistance." *PLoS ONE* 5, no. 9 (2010): e12875.

Ardern, K. D. and Ram, F. S. "Tartrazine Exclusion for Allergic Asthma." *The Cochrane Database of Systematic Review* 4, (2001) DOI: 10.1002/14651858.CD000460

Aronne, L. J. "Treating Obesity: A New Target for Prevention of Coronary Heart Disease." *Progress in Cardiovascular Nursing* 16, no. 3 (2001): 98–106, 115, PMID: 11464439.

Arscott, S. A., Howe, J. A., Davis, C. R., and Tanumihardjo, S. A. "Carotenoid Profiles in Provitamin A-containing Fruits and Vegetables Affect the Bioefficacy in Mongolian Gerbils." *Experimental Biology and Medicine (Maywood)* 235, no. 7 (July 2010): 839–848, PMID: 20558838.

Aruna, K. and Sivaramakrishnan, V. M. "Plant Products as Protective Agents Against Cancer." *Indian Journal of Experimental Biology* 28, no. 11 (November 1990): 1008–1011, PMID: 2283166.

Aruna, K., Rukkumani, R., Varma, P. S., and Menon, V. P. "Therapeutic Role of *Cuminum Cyminum* on Ethanol and Thermally Oxidized Sunflower Oil Induced Toxicity." *Phytotherapy Research* 19, no. 5 (May 2005): 416–421, PMID: 16106395.

Attia, W. Y., Gabry, M. S., El-Shaikh, K. A., and Othman, G. A. "The Anti-Tumor Effect of Bee Honey in Ehrlich Ascite Tumor Model of Mice Is Coincided with Stimulation of the Immune Cells." *The Egyptian Journal of Immunology* 15, no. 2 (2008): 169–183, PMID: 20306700.

Avery, Jenna. "Eat Your Veggies, Raise Your Vibration." Living Your Purpose Blog. Accessed Mar 27, 2009. http://www.highlysensitivesouls.com/blog/?p=380.

Balandraud, N. and Roudier, J. "Epstein-Barr Virus and Rheumatoid Arthritis." *Joint Bone Spine* (2017): pii: S1297-319X(17)30093-3. PMID: 28499895.

Bammens, B., Verbeke, K., Vanrenterghem, Y., and Evenepoel, P. "Evidence for Impaired Assimilation of Protein in Chronic Renal Failure." *Kidney International* 64, no. 6 (December 2003): 2196–2203, PMID: 14633143.

Banner, W. P., DeCosse, J. J., Tan, Q. H., and Zedeck, M. S. "Selective Distribution of Selenium in Colon Parallels Its Antitumor Activity." *Carcinogenesis* 5, no. 12 (December 1984): 1543–1546, PMID: 6499107.

Bazzano, L. A., He, J., Odgen, L. G., Loria, C., Vupputuri, S., Myers, L., and Whelton, P. K. "Dietary Intake of Folate and Risk of Stroke in US Men and Women: NHANES I Epidemiologic Follow-Up Study." *Stroke* 33, no. 5 (May 2002): 1183–1189.

Bengtsson, A., Larsson-Alminger, M., and Svanberg, U. "In Vitro Bioaccessibility of Beta-Carotene from Heat-Processed Orange-Fleshed Sweet Potato." *Journal of Agricultural and Food Chemistry* 57, no. 20 (October 2009): 9693–9698, PMID: 19807125.

Benmassaoud, A., McDonald, E. G., and Lee, T. C. "Potential Harms of Proton Pump Inhibitor Therapy: Rare Adverse Effects of Commonly Used Drugs." *Canadian Medical Association Journal* 188, no. 9 (June 2015): 657–62.

Bennett, A., Bending, G., Chandler, D., Hilton, S., and Mills, P. "Meeting the Demand for Crop Production: The Challenge of Yield Decline in Crops Grown in Short Rotations." *Biological Reviews* 87, no. 1 (2012): 52–71.

Benyesh-Melnick, M., Rosenberg, H. S., and Watson, B. "Viruses in Cell Cultures of Kidneys of Children with Congenital Heart Malformations and Other Diseases." *Proceedings of the Society for Experimental Biology and Medicine* 117, no. 2 (1964): 452–459.

Best, R., Lewis, D. A., and Nasser, N. "The Antiulcerogenic Activity of the Unripe Plantain Banana (Musa Species)." *British Journal of Pharmacology* 82, no. 2 (1984): 107–116.

Berenguer, T., Jakszyn, P., Barricarte, A., Ardanaz, E., Amiano, P., Dorronsoro, M., Larrañaga, N., et al. "Estimation of Dietary Sources and Flavonoid Intake in a Spanish Adult Population (EPIC-Spain)." *Journal of the American Dietetic Association* 110, no. 3 (March 2010): 390, PMID: 20184989.

Blomhoff, R., Carlsen, M. H., Andersen, L. F., and Jacobs, D. R. Jr. "Health Benefits of Nuts: Potential Role of Antioxidants." *British Journal of Nutrition* 96, no. 2 (November 2006): S52–S60, PMID: 17125534.

Boué, S. M., Wiese, T. E., Nehls, S., Burow, M. E., Elliott, S., Carter-Wientjes, C. H., Shih, B. Y., et. al. "Evaluation of the Estrogenic Effects of Legume Extracts Containing Phytoestrogens." *Journal of Agricultural and Food Chemistry* 51, no. 8 (April 2003): 2193–2199, PMID: 12670155.

Bouhdid, S., Abrini, J., Amensour, M., Zhiri, A., Espuny, M. J., and Manresa, A. "Functional and Ultrastructural Changes in *Pseudomonas Aeruginosa* and Staphylococcus Aureus Cells Induced by *Cinnamomum Verum* Essential Oil." *Journal of Applied Microbiology* 109, no. 4 (April 2010): 1139–1149.

Brady, N. F., Molan, P. C., and Harfoot, C. G. "The Sensitivity of Dermatophytes to the Antimicrobial Activity of Manuka Honey and Other Honey." *Pharmacy and Pharmacology Communications* 2, no. 10 (1997): 1–3.

Broadhurst, C. L., Polansky, M. N, and Anderson, R. A. "Insulin-like Biological Activity of Culinary and Medicinal Plant Aqueous Extracts in Vitro." Journal of Agricultural and Food Chemistry 48, no. 3 (2000): 849.

Burger, J., Stern, A. H., and Gochfeld, M. "Mercury in Commercial Fish: Optimizing Individual Choices to Reduce Risk." Environmental Health Perspectives 113, no. 3 (March 2005): 266–271, PMID: 15743713; PMCID: PMC1253750.

Burk, D. R., Senechal-Willis, P., Lopez, L. C., Hogue, B. G., and Daskalova, S. M. "Suppression of Lipopolysaccharide-Induced Inflammatory Responses in RAW 264. 7 Murine Macrophages by Aqueous Extract of *Clinopodium Vulgare L. (Lamiaceae)*." Journal of Ethnopharmacology 126, no. 3 (December 2009): 397–405, PMID: 19770031.

Byrnes, A. E., Lee, J. L., Brighton, R. E., Leeds, A.R., Dornhorst, A., and Frost G.S. "A Low Glycemic Diet Significantly Improves the 25-h Blood Glucose Profile in People with Type 2 Diabetes, Assessed Using the Continuous Glucose MiniMed Monitor." Diabetes Care 26 (2003): 548–549.

Caldwell, C. R. "Oxygen Radical Absorbance Capacity of the Phenolic Compounds in Plant Extracts Fractionated by High-Performance Liquid Chromatography." Analytical Biochemistry 293, no. 2 (June 2001): 232–238, PMID: 11399037.

Calkin, C. V. and Carandang, C. G. "Certain Eating Disorders May Be a Neuropsychiatric Manifestation of PANDAS: Case Report." Journal of the Canadian Academy of Child and Adolescent Psychiatry 16, no. 3 (2007): 132–135.

Canene-Adams, K., Lindshield, B. L., Wang, S., Jeffery, E. H., Clinton, S. K., and Erdman, J. W. Jr. "Epidemiology and Prevention Combinations of Tomato and Broccoli Enhance Antitumor Activity in Dunning R3327-H Prostate Adenocarcinomas." Cancer Research 67, no. 2 (2007): 836–843.

Cao, H., Urban, J. F. Jr., and Anderson, R. A. "Cinnamon Polyphenol Extract Affects Immune Responses by Regulating Anti- and Proinflammatory and Glucose Transporter Gene

Expression in Mouse Macrophages." The Journal of Nutrition 138, no. 5 (May 2008): 833–840, PMID: 18424588.

Cardoso, C. R., Favoreto, S. Jr., Oliveira, L. L., Vancim, J. O., Barban, G. B., Ferraz, D. B., Silva, J. S. "Oleic Acid Modulation of the Immune Response in Wound Healing: A New Approach for Skin Repair." Immunobiology 216, no. 3 (2011): 409–415, PMID: 20655616.

Carter, C. J. "Alzheimer's Disease: A Pathogenetic Autoimmune Disorder Caused by Herpes Simplex in a Gene-Dependent Manner." International Journal of Alzheimer's Disease (December 2010): 140539. http://dx.doi.org/10.4061/2010/140539.

Cassat, J. E. and Skaar, E. P. "Iron in Infection and Immunity." Cell Host & Microbe 13, no. 5 (2013): 509–519.

Cascarina, S.M. and Ross, E.D. "Yeast Prions and Human Prion-Like Proteins: Sequence Features and Prediction Methods." Cellular and Molecular Life Sciences 71, no. 11 (2014): 2047–2063.

Centers for Disease Control and Prevention (CDC). "National Diabetes Fact Sheet 2007 Figure Descriptions." Accessed on August 8, 2010. http://www.cdc.gov/diabetes/pubs/figuretext07.htm.

Ceballos-Marquez, A., Barkema, H. W., Stryhn, H., Wichtel, J. J., Neumann, J., Mella, A., Kruze, J., Espindola, M. S., and Wittwer, F. "The Effect of Selenium Supplementation Before Calving on Early-Lactation Udder Health in Pastured Dairy Heifers." Journal of Dairy Science 93, no. 10 (October 2010): 4602–4612, PMID: 20854994.

Center for Celiac Disease Research: University of Maryland School of Medicine. University of Maryland School of Medicine. Accessed January 26, 2018. http://www.massgeneral.org/children/services/treatmentprograms.aspx?id=1723&display=patient-education.

Chandalia, M., Garg, A., Lutjohann, D., von Bergmann, K., Grundy, S. M., and Brinkley, L. J. "Beneficial effects of High Dietary Fiber Intake in Patients with Type 2 Diabetes Mellitus." The New England Journal of Medicine 342, no. 19 (2002): 1392–1398.

Chavan, J. K., Kadam, S. S., and Salunkhe, D. K. "Biochemistry and Technology of Chickpea (*Cicer Arietinum L.*) Seeds." Critical Reviews in Food Science and Nutrition 25, no. 2 (1986): 107–158.

Chen, W., Duizer, L., Corredig, M., and Goff, H. D. "Addition of Soluble Soybean Polysaccharides to Dairy Products as a Source of Dietary Fiber." Journal of Food Science 75, no. 6 (August 2010): C478–C484, PMID: 20722900.

Chinni, S. R., Li, Y., Upadhyay, S., Koppolu, P. K., and Sarkar, F. H. "Indole-3-Carbinol (I3C) Induced Cell Growth Inhibition, G1 Cell Cycle Arrest and Apoptosis in Prostate Cancer Cells." *Oncogene* 20, no. 23 (May 2001): 2927–2936, PMID: 11420705.

Chiti, F. and Dobson, C. M. "Protein Misfolding, Functional Amyloid, and Human Disease." *Annual Review of Biochemistry* 75 (2006): 333–66.

Ciryam, P., Tartaglia, G. G., Morimoto, R. I., Dobson, C. M., and Vendruscolo, M. "Widespread Aggregation and Neurodegenerative Diseases are Associated with Supersaturated Proteins." *Cell Reports* 5, no. 3 (2013): 781–790.

Cogan T. A., Thomas A. O., Rees, L. E., Taylor A. H., Jepson M. A., Williams P. H., Ketley J., and Humphrey T. J. "Norepinephrine Increases the Pathogenic Potential of Campylobacter Jejuni." *Gut* 56, no. 8 (August 2007): 1060–1065.

Cohen, J. H., Kristal, A. R., and Stanford, J. L. "Fruit and Vegetable Intakes and Prostate Cancer Risk." *Journal of the National Cancer Institute* 92, no. 1 (January 2000): 61–68, PMID: 10620635.

Cohen, Suzy. "Methylation Problems Lead to 100s of Diseases." Suzy Cohen: America's Most Trusted Pharmacist. Accessed January 27, 2018. https://suzycohen.com/articles/methylation-problems/.

Collett, E. D., Davidson, L. A., Fan, Y. Y., Lupton, J. R., and Chapkin, R. S. "N-6 and N-3 Polyunsaturated Fatty Acids Differentially Modulate Oncogenic Ras Activation in Colonocytes." *American Journal of Physiology—Cell Physiology* 280, no. 5 (May 2001): C1066–C1075, PMID: 11287318.

Cook, L. C., LaSarre, B., and Federle, M. J. "Interspecies Communication Among Commensal and Pathogenic Streptococci." *mBio* 4, no. 4 (2013): e00382–13, http://doi.org/10.1128/mBio.00382-13.

Côté, J., Caillet, S., Doyon, G., Sylvain, J. F., and Lacroix, M. "Bioactive Compounds in Cranberries and Their Biological Properties." Critical Reviews in Food Science and Nutrition 50, no. 7 (August 2010): 666–679, PMID: 20694928.

Council for Agricultural Science and Technology (CAST). "Mycotoxins: Economic and Health Risks." *CAST: The Science Source for Food, Agricultural, and Environmental Issues*, December 1989. http://www.cast-science.org/publications/?mycotoxins_economic_and_health_risks=&show=product&productID=2869.

Cowan, D. F., and Johnson, W.C. "Amyloidosis in the White Pekin Duck. I. Relation to Social Environmental Stress." *Laboratory Investigation* 23 (1970): 551–555.

Cozzi, P.J., Abu-Jawdeh, G. M., Green, R. M., and Green, D. "Amyloidosis in Association with Human Immunodeficiency Virus Infection." *Clinical Infectious Diseases: An Official Publication of the Infectious Diseases Society of America* 14, no. 1 (1992): 189–91.

Crujeiras, A. B, Parra, D., Abete, I., and Martínez, J. A. "A Hypocaloric Diet Enriched in Legumes Specifically Mitigates Lipid Peroxidation in Obese Subjects." *Free Radical Research* 41, no. 4 (January 2007): 498–506.

Cui, D., Kawano, H., Hoshii, Y., Liu, Y. and Ishihara, T. "Acceleration of Murine AA Amyloid Deposition by Bovine Amyloid Fibrils and Tissue Homogenates." *Amyloid* 15, no. 2 (2008): 77–83.

Cui, D., Kawano, H., Takahashi, M., Hoshii, Y., Setoguchi, M., Gondo, T. and Ishihara, T. "Acceleration of Murine AA Amyloidosis by Oral Administration of Amyloid Fibrils Extracted from Different Species." *Pathology International* 52, no. 1 (2002): 40–45.

Cutler, G. J., Nettleton, J. A., Ross, J. A., Harnack, L. J., Jacobs, D. R., Scrafford, C. G., Barraj, L. M., Mink, P. J., and Robien, K. "Dietary Flavonoid Intake and Risk of Cancer in Postmenopausal Women: The Iowa Women's Health Study." *International Journal of Cancer* 123, no. 3 (August 2008): 664–671.

Czerwiski, J., Bartnikowska, E., Leontowicz, H., Lange, E., Leontowicz, M., Katrich, E., Trakhtenberg, S., and Gorinstein, S. "Oat (*Avena Sativa L.*) and Amaranth (*Amaranthus Hypochondriacus*) Meals Positively Affect Plasma Lipid Profile in Rats Fed Cholesterol-Containing Diets." *The* Journal of Nutriti*onal Biochemistry* 15, no. 10 (October 2004): 622–629, PMID: 15542354.

Davidson, B., Maciver, J., Lessard, E., and Connors, K. "Meat Lipid Profiles: A Comparison of Meat from Domesticated and Wild Southern African Animals." *In Vivo* 25, no. 2 (2011): 197–202.

Demirkaya, S., Vural, O., Dora, B., and Topcuoglu, M. A. "Efficacy of Intravenous Magnesium Sulfate in the Treatment of Acute Migraine Attacks." *Headache* 41, no. 2 (2001): 171–177.

DeToma, A.S., Salamekh, S., Ramamoorthy. A., and Lim, M.H. "Misfolded Proteins in Alzheimer's Disease and Type 2 Diabetes." *Chemical Society Reviews* 41, no. 2 (2012): 608–621.

Ding, H., Chin, Y. W., Kinghorn, A. D., and D'Ambrosio, S. M. "Chemopreventive Characteristics of Avocado Fruit." *Seminar in Cancer Biology* 17, no. 5 (May 2007): 386–394, PMID: 17582784.

Divis, D., Di Tommaso, S., Salvemini, S., Garramone, M., and Crisci, R. "Diet and Cancer." *Acta BioMedica* 77, no. 2 (August 2006): 118–123.

Donohue, M. J. "Sulfur Part I: Sulfur and Sulfur Compounds in the Environment." Accessed January 29, 2017. http://www.toxipedia.org/display/toxipedia/Mark+J++Donohue.

Donohue, M. J. "Sulfur Part II: Sulfur and Sulfur Compounds in the Human Body." Accessed January 29, 2017. http://www.toxipedia.org/display/toxipedia/Mark+J++Donohue.

Donohue, M. J. "The Detoxification System Part III: Sulfoxidation and Sulfation." Accessed January 29, 2017. http://www.toxipedia.org/display/toxipedia/Mark+J++Donohue.

Draper, C. R., Edel, M. J., Dick, I. M., Randall, A. G., Martin, G. B., and Prince, R. L. "Phytoestrogens Reduce Bone Loss and Bone Resorption in Oophorectomized Rats." The Journal of Nutrition 127, no. 9 (September 1997): 1795–1799.

Dreyfuss, J. L., Regatieri, C. V., Lima, M. A., Paredes-Gamero, E. J., Brito, A. S., Chavante, S. F., Belfort, R., Farah, M. E., and Nader, H. B. "A Heparin Mimetic Isolated from a Marine Shrimp Suppresses Neovascularization." *Journal of Thrombosis and Haemostasis* 8, no. 8: (May 2010): 1828-1837. PMID: 20492474.

Dubois, J., Ismail, A. A., Chan, S. L., and Ali-Khan, Z. "Fourier Transform Infrared Spectroscopic Investigation of Temperature- and Pressure-Induced Disaggregation of Amyloid A." *Scandinavian Journal of Immunology* 49, no. 4 (1999): 376–380.

Dunn, B. K., Richmond, E. S., Minasian, L. M., Ryan, A. M., and Ford, L. G. "A Nutrient Approach to Prostate Cancer Prevention: The Selenium and Vitamin E Cancer Prevention Trial (SELECT)." *Nutrition and Cancer* 62, no. 7 (October 2010): 896–918, PMID: 20924966.

Eberhardt, M. V., Kobira, K., Keck, A. S., Juvik, J. A., and Jeffery, E. H. "Correlation Analyses of Phytochemical Composition, Chemical, and Cellular Measures of Antioxidant Activity of Broccoli (*Brassica Oleracea L. Var. Italica*)." Journal of Agricultural and Food Chemistry 53, no. 19 (2005): 7421–7431, PMID: d16159168.

Egmond, H. P. and Jonker, M. A. *Worldwide Regulations for Mycotoxin in Foods and Feeds in 2003*. Rome, Italy: Food and Agriculture Organization of the United Nations, 2004.

El-Adawy, T. A. "Nutritional Composition and Antinutritional Factors of Chickpeas (*Cicer Arietinum L.*) Undergoing Different Cooking Methods and Germination." *Plant Foods for Human Nutrition* 57, no. 1 (2002): 83–97. PMID: 11855623.

Emery, P., Bradley, H., Arthur, V., Tunn, E., and Waring, R. "Genetic Factors Influencing the Outcome of Early Arthritis—The Role of Sulphoxidation Status." *British Journal of Rheumatology* 31, no. 7 (July 1992): 449–51.

Enewold, L., Zhu, K., Ron, E., Marrogi, A. J., Stojadinovic, A., Peoples, G. E., and Devesa, S. S. "Rising Thyroid Cancer Incidence in the United States by Demographic and Tumor Characteristics, 1980-2005." *Cancer Epidemiology and Prevention Biomarkers* 18, no. 3 (2009): 784–791.

Ensminger, A. H. Food for Health: A Nutrition Encyclopedia. Clovis, California: Pegus Press, 1986.

Esquenazi, D., Wigg, M. D., Miranda, M. M., Rodrigues, H. M., Tostes, J. B., Rozental, S., Da Silva, A. J. and Alviano, C. S. "Antimicrobial and Antiviral Activities of Polyphenolics from Cocos Nucifera Linn. (Palmae) Husk Fiber Extract." *Research in Microbiology* 153, no. 10 (December 2002): 647–652, PMID: 12558183.

Environmental Working Group. EWG's Shopper's Guide to Pesticides. Washington D.C.: FAO (Food and Agriculture Organization) (2004) Accessed January 29, 2018. https://www.ewg.org/foodnews/#.WmssIEmWzcu.

Feder, H. M. Jr., Gerber, M. A., Luger, S. W, and Ryan, R. W. "False-Positive Serologic Tests for Lyme Disease After Varicella Infection." The New England Journal of Medicine 325 (1991): 1886-7.

Fernandez, S. V. and Russo, J. "Estrogen and Xenoestrogens in Breast Cancer." *Toxicology Pathology* 38, no. 1 (2010): 110–122, PMID: 19933552.

Fielding, J. M., Rowley, K. G., Cooper, P., and O'Dea, K. "Increases in Plasma Lycopene Concentration After Consumption of Tomatoes Cooked with Olive Oil." *Asia Pacific Journal of Clinical Nutrition* 14, no. 2 (2005): 131–136, PMID: 15927929.

Fischer, L. M., daCosta, K. A., Kwock, L., Stewart, P. W., Lu, T. S., Stabler, S. P., Allen, R. H., and Zeisel, S. H. "Sex and Menopausal Status Influence Human Dietary Requirements for the Nutrient Choline." *The American Journal of Clinical Nutrition* 85, no. 5 (May 2007): 1275–1285, PMID: 17490963.

Fitzpatrick, M. "Soy Formulas and the Effects of Isoflavones on the Thyroid." *The New Zealand Medical Journal* 113, no. 1103 (February 2011): 24–26, PMID: 11482324.

Food Intolerance Institute of Australia. "Food Intolerance (Food Sensitivity)." Accessed January 26, 2018. http://www.foodintol.com/food_intolerance/ food_ intolerance.htm.

Fukushima, C., Matsuse, H., Tomari, S., Obase, Y., Miyazaki, Y., Shimoda, T., and Kohno, S. "Oral Candidiasis Associated with Inhaled Corticosteroid Use: Comparison of Fluticasone and Beclomethasone." *Annals of Allergy, Asthma, & Immunology* 90, no. 6 (June 2003): 646–651, PMID: 12839324.

Gabrovska, D., Fiedlerova, V., Holasova, M., Masková, E., Smrcinov, H., Rysová, J., Winterová, R., Michalová, A, Hutar, M. "The Nutritional Evaluation of Underutilized Cereals and Buckwheat." *Food and Nutrition Bulletin* 23, no. 3 (2002): 246–249.

Gallo, P. M., Rapsinski, G. J., Wilson, R. P., Oppong, G. O., Sriram, U., Goulian, M., Buttaro, B., Caricchio, R., Gallucci, S., and Tükel, Ç. "Amyloid-DNA Composites of Bacterial Biofilms Stimulate Autoimmunity." *Immunity* 42, no. 6 (2015): 1171–1184.

Gastaminza, G., Quirce, S., Torres, M., Tabar, A., Echechipía, S., Muñoz, D., and Fernández de Corres, L. "Pickled Onion-Induced Asthma: A Model of Sulfite-Sensitive Asthma?" *Allergy* 25, no. 8 (August 1995): 698–703, PMID: 7584680.

Giacco, R., Parillo, M., Rivellese, A. A., Lasorella, G., Giacco, A., D'episcopo, L., and Riccardi, G. "Long-Term Dietary Treatment with Increased Amounts of Fiber-Rich Low-Glycemic Index Natural Foods Improves Blood Glucose Control and Reduces the Number of Hypoglycemic Events in Type 1 Diabetic Patients." Diabetes Care 23, no. 10 (2000): 1461–1466.

Gidalevitz, T., Ben-Zvi, A., Ho, K. H., Brignull, H. R., and Morimoto, R. I. "Progressive Disruption of Cellular Protein Folding in Models of Polyglutamine Diseases." *Science* 311, no. 5766 (2006): 1471–1474.

Goel, A. and Aggarwal, B. B. "Curcumin, the Golden Spice from Indian Saffron, is a Chemosensitizer and Radiosensitizer for Tumors and Chemoprotector and Radioprotector for Normal Organs." *Nutrition and Cancer* 62, no. 7 (October 2010): 919–930, PMID: 20924967.

Golden, E. B., Lam, P. Y., Kardosh, A., Gaffney, K. J., Cadenas, E., Louie, S. G., Petasis, N. A., Chen, T. C., and Schonthal A. H. "Green Tea Polyphenols Block the Anticancer Effects of Bortezomib and Other Boronic Acid-Based Proteasome Inhibitors." *Blood* 113, no. 23 (June 2009): 5927–5937.

González-Périz, A., Horrillo, R., Ferré, N., Gronert, K., Dong, B., Morán-Salvador, E., Titos, E., et al. "Obesity-Induced Insulin Resistance and Hepatic Steatosis Are Alleviated by Omega-3 Fatty Acids: A Role for Resolvins and Protectins." *FASEB Journal* 23, no. 6 (June 2009): 1946–1957, PMID: 19211925; PMCID: PMC2698663.

Goossens, H.A., Nohlmans, M. K., and van den Bogaard, A. E. "Epstein-Barr Virus and Cytomegalovirus Infections Cause False-Positive Results in IgM Two-Test Protocol for Early Lyme Borreliosis." *Infection* 27, no. 3 (1999): 231.

Gragnoli, C. "Hypothesis of the Neuroendocrine Cortisol Pathway Gene Role in the Comorbidity of Depression, Type 2 Diabetes, and Metabolic Syndrome." *The Application of Clinical Genetics* 7, (2014): 43–53.

Greger, M. "Amyloid Fibrils: Potential Food Safety Implications." *International Journal of Food Safety, Nutrition and Public Health* 1, no. 2 (January 2008): 103–15.

Griel, A. E. and Kris-Etherton, P. M. "Tree Nuts and the Lipid Profile: A Review of Clinical Studies." The British Journal of Nutrition 96, no. 2 (November 2006): S68-S78, Erratum in: The British Journal of Nutrition 99, no. 2 (February 2008): 447-448, PMID: 17125536.

Gullett, N. P., Ruhul-Amin, A. R., Bayraktar, S., Pezzuto, J. M., Shin, D. M., Khuri, F. R., Aggarwal, B. B., Surh, Y. J., and Kucuk, O. "Cancer Prevention with Natural Compounds." *Seminars in Oncology* 37, no. 3 (June 2010): 258–281, PMID: 20709209.

Haenisch, B., von Holt, K., Wiese, B., Prokein, J., Lange, C., Ernst, A., Brettschneider, C., et al. "Risk of Dementia in Elderly Patients with the Use of Proton Pump Inhibitors." *European Archives of Psychiatry and Clinical Neuroscience* 265 no. 5, (2015): 419–28.

Hammer, K. A., Carson, C. F., and Riley, T. V. "Antimicrobial Activity of Essential Oils and Other Plant Extracts." Journal of Applied Microbiology 6, no. 6 (June 1999): 985–990, PMID: 10438227.

Hanson, J.D., Hendrickson, J., and Archer, D. "Challenges for Maintaining Sustainable Agricultural Systems in the United States." *Renewable Agriculture and Food Systems* 23, no. 4 (2008): 325–334.

Harris, S. A. and Harris, E. A. "Herpes Simplex Virus Type 1 and Other Pathogens are Key Causative Factors in Sporadic Alzheimer's Disease." *Journal of Alzheimer's Disease* 48, no. 2 (2015): 319–353, http://doi.org/10.3233/JAD-142853.

Haselkorn, T., Stewart, S. L., and Horn-Ross, P. L. "Why Are Thyroid Cancer Rates so High in Southeast Asian Women Living in the United States? The Bay Area Thyroid Cancer Study." *Cancer Epidemiology Biomarkers & Prevention* 12, no. 2 (February 2003): 144–150, PMID: 12582024.

Hashim, S. A., Clancy, R. E., Hegsted, D. M., and Stare, F. J. "Effect of Mixed Fat Formula Feeding on Serum Cholesterol Level in Man." *The American Journal of Clinical Nutrition* 7, no. 1 (1959): 30–34.

Häusler, M., Ramaekers, V. T., Doenges, M., Schweizer, K., Ritter, K., and Schaade, L. "Neurological Complications of Acute and Persistent Epstein-Barr Virus Infection in Paediatric Patients." *Journal of Medical Virology* 68, no. 2 (October 2002): 253–63.

He, M., van Dam, R. M., Rimm, E., Hu, F. B., and Qi, L. "Whole-Grain, Cereal Fiber, Bran, and Germ Intake and the Risks of All-Cause and Cardiovascular Disease-Specific Mortality Among Women with Type 2 Diabetes Mellitus." *Circulation* 121, no. 20 (May 2010): 2162–2168, PMID: 20458012; PMCID: PMC2886277.

Head, K. A. and Kelly, G. S. "Nutrients and Botanicals for Treatment of Stress: Adrenal Fatigue, Neurotransmitter Imbalance, Anxiety, and Restless Sleep." *Alternative Medicine Review* 14, no. 2 (June 2009): 114–140, PMID: 19594222.

"Health Benefits of Sheep's Milk." Ovis Angelica Divine Sheep's Cheese. Accessed September 1, 2010. http://www.sasheepdairy.co.za/benefits.html.

Hendrickson, John. "Energy Use in the U.S. Food System: A Summary of Existing Research and Analysis." Sustainable Farming-REAP-Canada 7, no. 4 (Fall 1996). Accessed January 29, 2018. https://www.cias.wisc.edu/wp-content/uploads/2008/07/energyuse.pdf.

Higgins, C. A., Bell, T., Delbederi, Z., Feutren-Burton, S., McClean, B., O'Dowd, C., Watters, W., Armstrong, P., Waugh, D., and van den Berg, H. "Growth Inhibitory Activity of Extracted Material and Isolated Compounds from the Fruits of *Kigelia Pinnata*." *Planta Medica* 76, no. 16 (November 2010): 1840-1846, PMID: 20560113.

Hinedi, T. B. and Koff, R. S. "Cholestatic Hepatitis Induced by Epstein-Barr Virus Infection in an Adult." *Digestive Diseases and Sciences* 48, no. 3 (March 2003): 539–41.

Hino, R., Uozaki, H., Murakami, N., Ushiku, T., Shinozaki, A., Ishikawa, S., and Morikawa, T. "Activation of DNA Methyltransferase 1 by EBV Latent Membrane Protein 2A Leads to Promoter Hypermethylation of PTEN Gene in Gastric Carcinoma." Cancer Research 69, no. 7 (April 2009): 2766–74.

Hlebowicz, J., Darwiche, G., Björgell, O., and Almér, L. O. "Effect of Cinnamon on Postprandial Blood Glucose, Gastric Emptying, and Satiety in Healthy Subjects." *The American Journal of Clinical Nutrition* 85, no. 6 (June 2007): 1552–1556.

Hossain, M. A., Kabir, M. J., Salehuddin, S. M., Rahman, S. M., Das, A. K., Singha, S. K., Alam, M. K., and Rahman, A. "Antibacterial Properties of Essential Oils and Methanol Extracts of Sweet Basil *Ocimum Basilicum* Occurring in Bangladesh." *Pharmaceutical Biology* 48, no. 5 (May 2010): 504–511.

Hou, W. C., Chen, Y. C., Chen, H. J., Lin, Y.H., Yang, L.L., and Lee, M.H. "Antioxidant Activities of Trypsin Inhibitor, a 33 KDa Root Storage Protein of Sweet Potato (*Ipomoea Batatas (L.)* Lam cv. Tainong 57)." Journal of Agricultural and Food Chemistry 49, no. 6 (June 2001): 2978–2981, PMID: 13860.

Hsu, J. C., Zhang, J., Dev, A., Wing, A., Bjeldanes, L. F., and Firestone, G. L. "Indole-3-Carbinol Inhibition of Androgen Receptor Expression and Downregulation of Androgen Responsiveness in Human Prostate Cancer Cells." Carcinogenesis 26, no. 11 (November 2005): 1896–1904. https://doi.org/10.1093/carcin/bgi155.

Hu, R., Khor, T. O., Shen, G., Jeong, W. S., Hebbar, V., Chen, C., Xu, C., Reddy, B., Chada, K., and Kong, A. N. "Cancer Chemoprevention of Intestinal Polyposis in ApcMin/+ Mice by Sulforaphane, a Natural Product Derived from Cruciferous Vegetable." *Carcinogenesis* 27, no. 10 (May 2006): 2038–2046, PMID: 16675473.

Hutt-Fletcher, L.M. "EBV Glycoproteins: Where Are We Now?" *Future Virol* 10, no. 10 (2015): 1155–1162.

Hwang, J. W., Jung, J. W., Lee, Y. S., and Kang, K. S. "Indole-3-Carbinol Prevents H(2)O(2)-Induced Inhibition of Gap Junctional Intercellular Communication by Inactivation of PKB/Akt." *The Journal of Veterinary Medical Science* 70, no. 10 (October 2008): 1057–1063, PMID: 18981661.

Hwang, S. Y., Siow, Y. L., Au-Yeung, K. K., House, J., and O. K. "Folic Acid Supplementation Inhibits NADPH Oxidase-Mediated Superoxide Anion Production in the Kidney." *American Journal of Physiology: Renal Physiology* 300, no. 1 (October 2010): F189–F198, PMID: 20980407.

Ibi, K., Murakami, T., Goda, W. M., Kobayashi, N., Ishiguro, N. and Yanal, T. "Prevalence of Amyloid Deposition in Mature Healthy Chickens in the Flock that Previously Had Outbreaks of Vaccine-Associated Amyloidosis." Journal of Veterinary Medical Science 77, no. 10 (2015): 1241–1245.

Islam, M. T. "Oxidative Stress and Mitochondrial Dysfunction-Linked Neurodegenerative Disorders." *Neurological Research* 39, no. 1 (January 2017): 73–82.

Ismail, M., Al-Naqeeb, G., Mamat, W. A., and Ahmad, Z. "Gamma-Oryzanol Rich Fraction Regulates the Expression of Antioxidant and Oxidative Stress Related Genes in Stressed Rat's Liver." *Nutrition and Metabolism (London)* 7, no. 23 (March 2010): 23, PMID: 20331906; PMCID: PMC2859356.

"Issues in a Nutshell: How Far Does Your Food Travel to Get to Your Plate?" CUESA, the Center for Urban Education about Sustainable Agriculture. Last modified September 20, 2010. http://www.cuesa.org/sustainable_ag/issues/foodtravel.php.

Jabeen, Q., Bashir, S., Lyoussi, B., and Gilani, A. H. "Coriander Fruit Exhibits Gut Modulatory, Blood Pressure Lowering and Diuretic Activities." Journal of Ethnopharmacology 122, no. 1 (February 2009): 123–130, PMID: 19146935.

Jacobs, D. R. Jr. and Gallaher, D. D. "Whole Grain Intake and Cardiovascular Disease: A Review." *Current Atherosclerosis Reports* 6, no. 6 (November 2004): 415–423, PMID: 15485586.

Jaga, K. and Brosius, D. "Pesticide Exposure: Human Cancers on the Horizon." *Rev Environ Health* 14, no. 1 (1999): 39–50.

Janegova, A., Janega, P., Rychly, B., Kuracinova, K., and Babal, P. "The Role of Epstein-Barr Virus Infection in the Development of Autoimmune Thyroid Diseases." *Endokrynologia Polska* 66, no. 2 (2015): 132–6.

Jang, D. S., Cuendet, M., Fong, H. H., Pezzuto, J., and Kinghorn, A. D. "Constituents of *Asparagus Officinalis* Evaluated for Inhibitory Activity Against Cyclooxygenase–2." Journal of Agricultural and Food Chemistry 52, no. 8 (2004): 2218–2222.

Jemai, H., Bouaziz, M., Fki, I., El Feki, A., and Sayadi, S. "Hypolipidimic and Antioxidant Activities of Oleuropein and Its Hydrolysis Derivative-Rich Extracts from *Chemlali Olive* Leaves." *Chemico-Biological Interactions* 176, no. 2-3 (2008): 88–98, PMID: 18823963.

Johnson-Winters, K., Tollin, G., and Enemark, J. H. "Elucidating the Catalytic Mechanism of Sulfite Oxidizing Enzymes Using Structural, Spectroscopic, and Kinetic Analyses." *Biochemistry* 49, no. 34 (August 2010): 7242–7254, PMID: 20666399; PMCID: PMC2927705.

Josse, A. R., Kendall, C. W., Augustin, L. S., Ellis, P. R., and Jenkins, D. J. "Almonds and Postprandial Glycemia—A Dose Response Study." *Metabolism* 56, no. 3 (March 2007): 400–404.

Jovanovic, A., Gerrard, J., and Taylor, R. "The Second-Meal Phenomenon in Type 2 Diabetes." Diabetes Care 32, no. 7 (July 2009): 1199–1201, PMID: 19366973; PMCID: PMC2699724.

Judith, K., Donnelly, D., and Robinson, S. "Invited Review Free Radicals in Foods Free Radical Research." *Free Radical Research* 2, no. 2 (January 1995): 147–176.

Kanter, M. M. "Free Radicals, Exercise, and Antioxidant Supplementation." *International Journal of Sport Nutrition* 4, no. 3 (September 1994): 205–220, PMID: 7987357.

Karadeniz, F., Durst, R. W., and Wrolstad, R. E. "Polyphenolic Composition of Raisins." Journal of Agricultural and Food Chemistry 48, no. 11 (November 2000): 5343–5350, PMID: 13500.

Kelm, M. A, Nair, M. G., Strasburg, G. M., and DeWitt, D. L. "Antioxidant and Cyclooxygenase Inhibitory Phenolic Compounds from *Ocimum Sanctum Linn*." *Phytomedicine* 7, no. 1 (March 2000): 7–13, PMID: 10782484.

Kendall, C. W., Esfahani, A., Truan, J., Srichaikul, K., and Jenkins, D. J. "Health Benefits of Nuts in Prevention and Management of Diabetes." *Asia Pacific Journal of Clinical Nutrition* 19, no. 1 (2010): 110–116, PMID: 20199995.

Khodavandi, A., Alizadeh, F., Aala, F., Sekawi, Z., and Chong, P. P. "In Vitro Investigation of Antifungal Activity of Allicin Alone and in Combination with Azoles against Candida Species." *Mycopathologia* 169, no. 4 (April 2010): 287–295, PMID: 19924565.

Khokhar, S. and Magnusdottir, S. G. "Total Phenol, Catechin, and Caffeine Contents of Teas Commonly Consumed in the United Kingdom." Journal of Agricultural and Food Chemistry 50, no. 3 (January 2002): 565–570.

Khoo, A. "Acute Cholestatic Hepatitis Induced by Epstein-Barr Virus Infection in an Adult: A Case Report." *Journal of Medical Case Reports* 10, no. 1 (March 2016): 75.

Knowles, T. P., Vendruscolo, M., and Dobson, C. M. "The Amyloid State and its Association with Protein Misfolding Diseases." *Nature Reviews: Molecular Cell Biology* 15, no. 6 (2014): 384–96.

Koga, H., Kaushik, S., and Cuervo, A. M. "Protein Homeostasis and Aging: The Importance of Exquisite Quality Control." *Ageing Research Reviews* 10, no. 2 (2011): 205–215.

Koop, C. E. "Surgeon General's Report 1988—Re Cholesterol." Accessed September 27, 2010. http://www.mcspotlight.org/media/reports/surgen_rep.html.

Koar, M., Dorman, H. J., Baer, K. H., and Hiltunen, R. "*Salvia Officinalis L.*: Composition and Antioxidant-Related Activities of a Crude Extract and Selected Sub-Fractions." *Natural Product Communications* 5, no. 9 (September 2010): 1453–1456, PMID: 20923007.

Kratzer, F. H., Williams, D. E., and Marshall, B. "The Tryptophan Requirement of Young Turkey Poults." The Journal of Nutrition 43, no. 2 (February 1952): 223–233, PMID: 14851040.

Kuipers, R. S., Smit, E. N., van der Meulen, J., Dijck-Brouwer, D. J., Boersma, E.R., and Muskiet, F. A. "Milk in the Island Of Chole [Tanzania] is High in Lauric, Myristic, Arachidonic and Docosahexaenoic Acids, and Low in Linoleic Acid Reconstructed Diet of Infants Born to Our Ancestors Living in Tropical Coastal Regions." *Prostaglandins Leukot Essent Fatty Acids* 76, no. 4 (April 2007): 221–233, PMID: 17383169.

Kung, J., Staub, R. E., Preobrazhenskaya, M. N., Bjeldanes, L. F., and Firestone, G. L. "1-Benzyl-Indole-3-Carbinol Is a Novel Indole-3-Carbinol Derivative with Significantly Enhanced Potency of Anti-Proliferative and Anti-Estrogenic Properties in Human Breast Cancer Cells." *Chemico-Biological Interactions* 186, no. 3 (August 2010): 255–266, PMID: 20570586.

Kushad, M. M., Brown, A. F., Kurilich, A. C., Juvik, J.A., Klein, B. P., Wallig, M. A., and Jeffery, E.H. "Variation of Glucosinolates in Vegetable Crops of Brassica Oleracea." Journal of Agricultural and Food Chemistry 47, no. 4 (April 1999): 1541–1548, PMID: 13320.

Lambert, R. J., Skandamis, P. M., Coote, P. J., and Nychas, G. J. "A Study of the Minimum Inhibitory Concentration and Mode of Action of Oregano Essential Oil, Thymol and Carvacol." Journal of Applied Microbiology 91, no. 3 (2001): 453–462.

Lammert, A., Kratzsch, J., Selhorst, J., Humpert, P. M., Bierhaus, A., Birck, R., Kusterer, K., and Hammes, H. P. "Clinical Benefit of a Short Term Dietary Oatmeal Intervention in Patients with Type 2 Diabetes and Severe Insulin Resistance: A Pilot Study." *Experimental and Clinical Endocrinology & Diabetes* 116, no. 2 (February 2008): 132–134, PMID: 18095234.

Lee, D. Y., Lee, D. G., Cho, J. G., Bang, M. H., Lyu, H. N., Lee, Y. H., Kim, S. Y., and Baek, N. I. "Lignans from the Fruits of the Red Pepper (*Capsicum Annuum L.*) and their Antioxidant

Effects." *Archives of Pharmacal Research* 32, no. 10 (October 2009): 1345–1349, PMID: 19898795.

Lee, J. S., Jeon, S. M., Park, E. M., Huh, T. L., Kwon, O. S., Lee, M. K., and Choi, M. S. "Cinnamate Supplementation Enhances Hepatic Lipid Metabolism and Antioxidant Defense Systems in High Cholesterol-Fed Rats." Journal of Medicinal Food 6, no. 3 (Fall 2003): 183–191, PMID: 14585184.

Leterme, P. "Recommendations by Health Organizations for Pulse Consumption." *The British Journal of Nutrition* 88, no. 3 (December 2002): S239–S242, PMID: 12498622.

Leung, E. H. and Ng, T. B. "A Relatively Stable Antifungal Peptide from Buckwheat Seeds with Antiproliferative Activity toward Cancer Cells." *Journal of Peptide Science 13*, no. 11 (November 2007): 762–767, PMID: 17828793.

Levitan, E. B., Wolk, A., and Mittleman, M. A. "Fatty Fish, Marine Omega-3 Fatty Acids and Incidence of Heart Failure." *European Journal of Clinical Nutrition* 64, no. 6 (June 2010): 587–594, PMID: 20332801.

"Liquid Chlorophyll—Alkaline By Design." Alkaline by Design. Accessed September 1, 2010. http://www.alkalinebydesign.co.uk/greens-powders-and-liquids/liquid-chlorophyll.

Lograda, T., Chaker, A. N., Chalchat, J. C., Ramdani, M., Silini, H., Figueredo, G., and Chalarde, P. "Chemical Composition and Antimicrobial Activity of Essential Oils of *Genista Ulicina* and *G. Vepres.*" *Natural Product Communications* 5, no. 5 (May 2010): 835–838.

Long, J., Gao, H., Sun, L., Liu, J., and Zhao-Wilson, X. "Grape Extract Protects Mitochondria from Oxidative Damage and Improves Locomotor Dysfunction and Extends Lifespan in a Drosophila Parkinson's Disease Model." *Rejuvenation Research* 12, no. 5 (October 2009): 321–331, PMID: 19929256.

Lonnerdal, B. "Dietary Factors Influencing Zinc Absorption." Journal of Nutrition 130, no. 5 (2000): 1378S–1383S.

López, L. R., Ledesma, A. C., Frati-Mjnari, B. C., Hernández-Domínguez, Cervantes, M. S., Hernandez, L. M., Juarez, C. and Moran, L. S. "Monounsaturated Fatty Acid (Avocado) Rich Diet for Mild Hypercholesterolemia." *Archives of Medical Research* 27, no. 4 (1996): 519–523.

López-López, A., Montaño, A., Cortés-Delgado, A., and Garrido-Fernández, A. "Survey of Vitamin B(6) Content in Commercial Presentations of Table Olives." *Plant Foods for Human Nutrition* 63, no. 2 (June 2008): 87–91, PMID: 18496754.

Lundmark, K., Westermark, G. T., Olsen, A., and Westermark, P. "Protein Fibrils in Nature Can Enhance Amyloid Protein A Amyloidosis in Mice: Cross-Seeding as a Disease Mechanism." *Proceedings of the National Academy of Sciences of the USA* 102, no. 17 (2005): 6098–102.

"Lung Cancer Associated with Beta-Carotene Supplementation in Smokers." *Prescrire International* 19, no. 107 (June 2010): 121, PMID: 20738040.

Lv, S., Fan, R., Du, Y., Hou, M., Tang, Z., Ling, W., and Zhu, H. "Betaine Supplementation Attenuates Atherosclerotic Lesion in Apolipoprotein E-Deficient Mice." *European* Journal of Nutrition 48, no. 4 (June 2009): 205–212, PMID: 19255798.

MacLea, K. S., "What Makes a Prion: Infectious Proteins from Animals to Yeast." *International Review of Cell and Molecular Biology* 329 (2017): 227–276.

Maekawa, A., Ogiu, T., Onodera, H., Furuta, K., Matsuoka, C., Ohno, Y., and Odashima, S. "Carcinogenicity Studies of Sodium Nitrite and Sodium Nitrate in F-344 Rats." *Food and Chemical Toxicology* 20, no. 1 (February 1982): 25–33, PMID: 7200054.

"Major Crops Grown in the United States—Ag 101—Agriculture—US EPA." The United States Environmental Protection Agency. Accessed September 14, 2010. http://www.epa.gov/agriculture/ag101/cropmajor.html.

Maiyoh, G. K., Kuh, J. E., Casaschi, A., and Theriault, A. G. "Cruciferous Indole-3-Carbinol Inhibits Apolipoprotein B Secretion in Hepg2 Cells." The Journal of Nutrition 137, no. 10 (October 2007): 2185–2189, PMID: 17884995.

Marconett, C. N., Sundar, S. N., Poindexter, K. M., Stueve, T. R., Bjeldanes, L. F., and Firestone, G. L. "Indole-3-Carbinol Triggers Aryl Hydrocarbon Receptor-Dependent Estrogen Receptor (ER) Alpha Protein Degradation in Breast Cancer Cells Disrupting an Eralpha-GATA3 Transcriptional Cross-Regulatory Loop." *Molecular Biology of the Cell* 21, no. 7 (April 2010): 1166–1177, PMID: 20130088.

Marler, J. B. and Wallin, J. R. "Human Health, the Nutritional Quality of Harvested Food and Sustainable Farming Systems." Nutrition Security Institute. Accessed January 29, 2018. https://content.siselinternational.com/sisel-int/science-pdfs/nutrition_triangleoflife.pdf.

Martínez, M. L., Labuckas, D. O., Lamarque, A. L., and Maestri, D. M. "Walnut (*Juglans Regia L.*): Genetic Resources, Chemistry, By-Products." Journal of the Science of Food and Agriculture 90, no. 12 (September 2010): 1959–1967, PMID: 20586084.

Martínez de Morentin, P. B., González, C. R., and López, M. "AMP-Activated Protein Kinase: 'A Cup of Tea' Against Cholesterol-Induced Neurotoxicity." *The Journal of Pathology* 222, no. 4 (September 2010): 329–334, PMID: 20922714.

Martinez-Tome, M., Jimenez, A. M., Ruggieri, S., Friga, N., Strabbioli, R., and Mercia, M. A. "Antioxidant Properties of Mediterranean Spices Compared with Common Food Additives." *Journal of Food Protection* 64, no. 9 (September 2001): 1412–1419. PMID: 12440.

Mas, S., Crescenti, A., Gassó, P., Deulofeu, R., Molina, R., Ballesta, A., Kensler, T. W., and Lafuente, A. "Induction of Apoptosis in HT-29 Cells by Extracts from Isothiocyanates-Rich Varieties of *Brassica Oleracea*." *Nutrition and Cancer* 58, no. 1 (2007): 107–14, PMID: 17571973.

Mattsson, N., Bremell, D., Anckarsäter, R., Blennow, K., Anckarsäter, H., Zetterberg, H., and Hagberg, L. "Neuroinflammation in Lyme Neuroborreliosis Affects Amyloid Metabolism." *BMC Neurology* 10 (2010): 51–56.

Maurer, H. R. "Bromelain: Biochemistry, Pharmacology and Medical Use." Cellular and Molecular Life Sciences 58, no. 9 (2001): 1234–1245.

Maury, W., Price, J. P., Brindley, M. A., Oh, C., Neighbors, J. D., Wiemer, D. F., Wills, N., et al. "Identification of Light-Independent Inhibition of Human Immunodeficiency Virus-1 Infection Through Bioguided Fractionation of *Hypericum Perforatum.*" *Virology Journal 6* (July 2009): 101.

McAfee, A. J., McSorley, E. M., Cuskelly, G. J., Fearon, A. M., Moss, B. W., Beattie, J. A., Wallace, J. M., Bonham, M. P., and Strain, J. J. "Red Meat from Animals Offered a Grass Diet Increases Plasma and Platelet N-3 PUFA in Healthy Consumers." *The British* Journal of Nutrition 105, no. 1 (September 2010): 80–89, PMID: 20807460.

Mendis, S., Samarajeewa, U., and Thattil, R. O. "Coconut Fat and Serum Lipoproteins: Effects of Partial Replacement with Unsaturated Fats." The British Journal of Nutrition 85, no. 5 (May 2001): 583–589, PMID: 11348573.

"Mercury Levels in Fish: American Pregnancy Association." Promoting Pregnancy Wellness: American Pregnancy Association. Accessed on September 27, 2010. http://www.americanpregnancy.org/pregnancyhealth/fishmercury.htm.

Mezuk, B., Eaton, W.W., Albrecht, S., and Golden, S. H. "Depression and Type 2 Diabetes Over the Lifespan: A Meta-Analysis." Diabetes Care 31, no. 12 (2008): 2383–2390.

Miklossy, J., Kis, A., Radenovic, A., Miller, L., Forro, L., Martins, R., Reiss, K., et al. "Beta-Amyloid Deposition and Alzheimer's Type Changes Induced By Borrelia Spirochetes." *Neurobiology of Aging* 27, no. 2 (2006): 228–236.

Miller, K. "Estrogen and DNA Damage: The Silent Source of Breast Cancer?" *Journal of the National Cancer Institute* 95, no. 2 (2003): 100–102.

Minton, Barbara. "Milk Destroys Antioxidant Benefits in Blueberries." Natural News.com: Natural Health, Natural Living, Natural News. Accessed February 3, 2009. http://www.naturalnews.com/025516_blueberries_antioxidant_cancer.html.

Miron, A., Hancianu, M., Aprotosoaie, A. C., Gacea, O., and Stanescu, U. "Contributions to Chemical Study of the Raw Polysaccharide Isolated from the Fresh Pressed Juice of White Cabbage Leaves." *Revista Medico-Chirugicala a Societatii de Medici si Naturalisti din Iasi* 110, no. 4 (October-December 2006): 1020–1026, PMID: 17438919.

Mittal, A., Ranganath, V., and Nichani, A. "Omega Fatty Acids and Resolution of Inflammation: A New Twist in an Old Tale." *Journal of Indian Society of Periodontology* 14, no. 1 (January 2010): 3–7, PMID: 20922071.

Mohan-Kumar, M., Joshi, M. C., Prabha, T., Dorababu, and M., Goel, R. K. "Effect of Plantain Banana on Gastric Ulceration in NIDDM Rats: Role of Gastric Mucosal Glycoproteins, Cell Proliferation, Antioxidants and Free Radicals." *Indian Journal of Experimental Biology* 44, no. 4 (2006): 292–299, PMID: 16629371.

Monroe, K. R., Murphy, S. P., Henderson, B. E., Kolonel, L. N., Stanczyk, F. Z., Adlercreutz, H., and Pike, M. C. "Dietary Fiber Intake and Endogenous Serum Hormone Levels in Naturally Postmenopausal Mexican American Women: The Multiethnic Cohort Study." *Nutrition and Cancer* 58, no. 2 (2007): 127–135.

Moon, D. O., Kim, M. O., Choi, Y. H., Park, Y. M., and Kim, G. Y. "Curcumin Attenuates Inflammatory Response in IL-1beta-Induced Human Synovial Fibroblasts and Collagen-Induced Arthritis in Mouse Model." *International Immunopharmacology* 10, no. 5 (May 2010): 605–610, PMID: 20188213.

Moreno-Gonzalez, I., Edwards III, G., Salvadores, N., Shahnawaz, M., Diaz-Espinoza, R., and Soto, C. "Molecular Interaction Between Type 2 Diabetes and Alzheimer's Disease Through Cross-Seeding of Protein Misfolding." *Molecular Psychiatry* 22, no. 9 (2017): 1327.

Moretti, A., Logrieco, A. F., and Susca, A. "Mycotoxins: An Underhand Food Problem." *Methods in Molecular Biology* 1542, (2017): 3–12.

Morris, G., Berk, M., Walder, K., and Maes, M. "The Putative Role of Viruses, Bacteria, and Chronic Fungal Biotoxin Exposure in the Genesis of Intractable Fatigue Accompanied by Cognitive and Physical Disability." *Molecular Neurobiology* 53, no. 4 (2016): 2550–2571.

Mukherjee, A., Morales-Scheihing, D., Salvadores, N., Moreno-Gonzalez, I., Gonzalez, C., Taylor-Presse, K., Mendez, N., et al. "Induction of IAPP Amyloid Deposition and Associated Diabetic Abnormalities by a Prion-Like Mechanism." *Journal of Experimental Medicine* 6, no. 23 (2017): 2591-2610, https://doi.org/10.1084/jem.20161134.

Munkvold, G. P. and Desjardins, A. E. "Fumonisins in Maize: Can We Reduce Their Occurrence?" *Plant Disease* 81 (1997): 556–565.

Munkvold, G. P. and Hellmich, R. L. "Comparison of Fumonisin Concentrations in Kernels of Transgenic Bt Maize Hybrids and Nontransgenic Hybrids." Plant Disease 83, no. 2 (1999):130–138.

Murakami, T., Inoshima, Y., Sakamoto, E., Fukushi, H., Sakai, H., Yanai, T., and Ishiguro, N. "AA Amyloidosis in Vaccinated Growing Chickens." *Journal of Comparative Pathology* 149, no. 2 (2013): 291-7.

Murakami, T., Ishiguro, N., and Higuchi, K. "Transmission of Systemic AA Amyloidosis in Animals." *Veterinary Pathology* 51, no. 2 (2014): 363–371.

Nahdi, A., Hammami, I., Kouidhi, W., Chargui, A., Ben-Ammar, A., Hamdaoui, M. H., El May, A., and El May, M. "Protective Effects of Crude Garlic by Reducing Iron-Mediated Oxidative Stress, Proliferation and Autophagy in Rats." *Journal of Molecular Histology* 41, no. 4–5 (October 2010): 233–245, PMID: 20700633.

Nakatsuji, T., Kao, M. C., Zhang, L., Zouboulis, C. C., Gallo, R. L., and Huang, C. M. "Sebum Free Fatty Acids Enhance the Innate Immune Defense of Human Sebocytes by Upregulating Beta-Defensin-2 Expression." *Journal of Investigative Dermatology* 130, no. 4 (April 2010): 985–994, PMID: 20032992.

Nater, U. M., La Marca, R., Florin, L., Moses, A., Langhans, W., Koller, M. M., and Ehlert, U. "Stress-Induced Changes in Human Salivary Alpha-Amylase Activity—Associations with Adrenergic Activity." Psychoneuroendocrinology 31, no. 1 (January 2006): 49–58, PMID: 16002223.

National Center for Health Statistics. "National Health and Nutrition Examination Survey (NHANES)." United States Department of Agriculture (USDA). Accessed November 1, 2016. https://www.cdc.gov/nchs/nhanes/index.htm.

Nejad, M. S. and Niroomand, A. "Study on Lipid Changes of Leaves and Fruits Olive Adapted to High Temperature Condition Inkhuzestan." Pakistan Journal of Biological Sciences 10, no. 24 (December 2017): 4535–4538, PMID: 19093527.

Nettleton, J. A. "Fatty Acids in Cultivated and Wild Fish." Presentation at the International Institute of Fisheries, Economics and Trade (IIFET) 2000 Conference: Microbehavior and Macroresults, Oregon State University, Corvallis, OR, July 10–14, 2000.

Neuhouser, M. L., Patterson, R. E., Thornquist, M. D. , Omen, G. S., King, I. B., and Goodman, G. E. "Fruits and Vegetables are Associated with Lower Lung Cancer Risk Only in the Placebo Arm of the Beta-Carotene and Retinol Efficacy Trial." *CARET* 12, no. 4 (2002): 350–358.

Neuman, H., Debelius, J. W., Knight, R., and Koren, O. "Microbial Endocrinology: The Interplay Between the Microbiota and the Endocrine System." *FEMS Microbiology Reviews* 39, no. 4 (2015): 509–521.

Nguyen, H. H., Lavrenov, S. N., Sundar, S. N., Nguyen, D. H., Tseng, M., Marconett, C. N., Kung, J., et al. "1-Benzyl-Indole-3-Carbinol is a Novel Indole-3-Carbinol Derivative with Significantly Enhanced Potency of Anti-Proliferative and Anti-Estrogenic Properties in Human Breast Cancer Cells." *Chemico-Biological Interactions* 186, 3 (August 2010): 255–266, PMID: 20570586.

Nicholas, J., Miller, M., and Ruiz-Larrea, B. "Flavonoids and Other Plant Phenols in the Diet: Their Significance as Antioxidants." Journal of Nutrition*al and Environmental Medicine* 12, no. 1 (January 2002): 39–51.

Nivsarkar, M. and Banerjee, A. "Establishing the Probable Mechanism of L-DOPA in Alzheimer's Disease Management." *Acta Poloniae Pharmaceutica* 66, no. 5 (September–October 2009): 483–486, PMID: 19894644.

Nyström, S. N. and Westermark, G. T. "AA-Amyloid is Cleared by Endogenous Immunological Mechanisms." *Amyloid* 19, no. 3 (2012): 138–145.

Ogungbenle, H. N. "Nutritional Evaluation and Functional Properties of Quinoa (*Chenopodium Quinoa*) Flour." *International Journal of Food Sciences and Nutrition* 54, no. 2 (2003): 153–158.

Olejnik, A., Tomczyk, J., Kowalska, K., and Grajek, W. "The Role of Natural Dietary Compounds in Colorectal Cancer Chemoprevention." *Postępy Higieny i Medycyny Doświadczalnej (Online)* 64 (April 2010): 175–187, PMID: 20400781.

Oli, M. W., Otoo, H. N., Crowley, P. J., Heim, K. P., Nascimento, M. M., Ramsook, C. B., Lipke, P. N. and Brady, L. J. "Functional Amyloid Formation by Streptococcus Mutans." *Microbiology* 158, no. 12 (2012): 2903–2916.

Ozgoli, G., Goli, M., and Simbar, M. "Effects of Ginger Capsules on Pregnancy, Nausea, and Vomiting." *Journal of Alternative and Complementary Medicine* 15, no. 3 (March 2009): 243–246, PMID: 19250006.

Pan, H. B., Zhao, X. L., Zhang, X., Zhang, K. B., Li, L. C., Li, Z. Y., Lam, W. M., et al. "Strontium Borate Glass: Potential Biomaterial for Bone Regeneration." *Journal of the Royal Society, Interface* 7, no. 48 (July 2010): 1025–1031, PMID: 20031984; PMCID: PMC2880081.

Pannellini, T., Iezzi, M., Liberatore, M., Sabatini, F., Iacobelli, S., Rossi, C., and Alberti, S. "A Dietary Tomato Supplement Prevents Prostate Cancer in TRAMP Mice." *Cancer Prevention Research (Philadelphia, Pa)* 3, no. 10 (August 2010): 1284–1291, PMID: 20716635.

Parker, Hilary. "A Sweet Problem: Princeton Researchers Find that High-Fructose Corn Syrup Prompts Considerably More Weight Gain." Princeton University. Last modified March 22, 2010. http://www.princeton.edu/main/news/archive/S26/91/22K07/.

Patel, V. B., Misra, S., Patel, B. B., and Majumdar, A. P. "Colorectal Cancer: Chemopreventive Role of Curcumin and Resveratrol." *Nutrition and Cancer* 62, no. 7 (October 2010): 958–967, PMID: 20924971.

Payne, G. A. "Process of Contamination by Aflatoxin-Producing Fungi and their Impact on Crops." *Mycotoxins in Agriculture and Food Safety* 9 (1998): 279–306.

Pellerin, P. "Goat's Milk in Nutrition." *Annales Pharmaceutiques Francaises* 59, no. 1 (2001): 51–62.

Penezić Z., Savić S., Vujović S., Tatić S., Ercegovac M., and Drezgićc M. "The Ectopic ACTH Syndrome." *Srp Arh Celok Lek* 132, no. 1–2 (2004): 28–32.

Percival, S. S., Talcott, S. T., Chin, S. T., Mallak, A. C., Lounds-Singleton, A., and Pettit-Moore, J. "Neoplastic Transformation of BALB/3T3 Cells and Cell Cycle Of HL-60 Cells Are Inhibited by Mango (*Mangifera Indica L.*) Juice and Mango Juice Extracts." The Journal of Nutrition 136, no. 5 (May 2006): 1300–1304, PMID: 16614420.

Petroianu, A., Alberti, L. R., Souza, S. D., and Martins, S. G. "Effect of Ascorbic Acid and Hidrocortisone on Intestinal Anastomotic Tension." *Revista do Colegio Brasileiro de Cirurgioes* 36, no. 6 (December 2009): 509–513, PMID: 20140395.

Phillips, K. "Plums Poised to Give Blueberries Run for the Money." AgriLife News. Last modified January 28, 2009. http://agnews.tamu.edu/showstory.php?id=950.

Ping, H., Zhang, G., and Ren, G. "Antidiabetic Effects of Cinnamon Oil in Diabetic KK-Ay Mice." *Food and Chemical Toxicology* 48, no. 8-9 (August-September 2010): 2344–2349.

Pittaway, J. K., Ahuja, K. D., Cehun, M., Chronopoulos, A., Robertson, I. K., Nestel, P. J., and Ball, M. J. "Dietary Supplementation with Chickpeas for at Least 5 Weeks Results in Small but

Significant Reductions in Serum Total and Low-Density Lipoprotein Cholesterols in Adult Women and Men." *Annals of Nutrition and Metabolism* 50, no. 6 (2006): 512–518, PMID: 17191025.

Pizzorno, Joseph E. and Murray, Michael T. *Textbook of Natural Medicine*. Missouri: Elsevier Health Sciences, 2013.

Nygård, O., Nordrehaug, J. E., Refsum, H., Ueland, P. M., Farstad, M. and Vollset, S. E., "Plasma Homocysteine Levels and Mortality in Patients with Coronary Artery Disease." *New England Journal of Medicine 337*, no. 4 (July 1997): 230–236.

Platel, K., Rao, A., Saraswathi, G., and Srinivasan, K. "Digestive Stimulant Action of Three Indian Spice Mixes in Experimental Rats." *Die Nahrung* 46, no. 6 (December 2002): 394–398, PMID: 12577586.

Plaza, L., Sánchez-Moreno, C., de Pascual-Teresa, S., de Ancos, B., and Cano, M. P. "Fatty Acids, Sterols, and Antioxidant Activity in Minimally Processed Avocados During Refrigerated Storage." Journal of Agricultural and Food Chemistry 57, no. 8 (April 2009): 3204–3209, PMID: 19278228.

Pollan, Michael. *The Omnivore's Dilemma: A Natural History of Four Meals*. New York: Penguin, 2006. 249–275.

Puertollano, M. A., de Pablo, M. A., and Alvarez de Cienfuegos, G. "Anti-Oxidant Properties of N-Acetyl-L-Cysteine Do Not Improve the Immune Resistance of Mice Fed Dietary Lipids to Listeria Monocytogenes Infection." *Clinical Nutrition* 22, no. 3 (June 2003): 313–319, PMID: 12765672.

Puig, J. G., Mateos, F. A., Miranda, M. E., Torres, R. J., de Miguel, E., Pérez de Ayala, C., and Gil, A. A. "Purine Metabolism in Women with Primary Gout." *The American Journal of Medicine* 97, no. 4 (October 1994): 332–338, PMID: 7942934.

Radek, M. and Savage, G. P. "Oxalates in Some Indian Green Leafy Vegetables." *International Journal of Food Sciences and Nutrition* 59, no. 3 (May 2008): 246–260, PMID: 18335334.

Raederstorff, D. "Antioxidant Activity of Olive Polyphenols in Humans: A Review." *International Journal for Vitamin and Nutrition Research* 79, no. 3 (May 2009): 152–165, PMID: 20209466.

Rai, D., Bhatia, G., Sen, T., and Palit, G. "Comparative Study of Perturbations of Peripheral Markers in Different Stressors in Rats." *Canadian Journal of Physiology and Pharmacology* 81, no. 12 (December 2003): 1139–1146, PMID: 14719033.

Rajaram, S., Burke, K., Connell, B., Myint, T., and Sabaté, J. "A Monounsaturated Fatty Acid-Rich Pecan-Enriched Diet Favorably Alters the Serum Lipid Profile of Healthy Men and Women." The Journal of Nutrition 131, no. 9 (September 2001): 2275–2279.

Ramoutar, R. R. and Brumaghim, J. L. "Antioxidant and Anticancer Properties and Mechanisms of Inorganic Selenium, Oxo-Sulfur, and Oxo-Selenium Compounds." *Cell Biochemistry and Biophysics* 58, no. 1 (July 2010): 1–23.

Reich, O., Regauer, S., and Scharf, S. "High Levels of Xenoestrogens in Patients with Low-Grade Endometrial Stromal Sarcoma—Report of Two Cases." *European Journal of Gynaecological Oncology* 31, no. 1 (2010): 105–106, PMID: 20349793.

Revell, P., Clark III, J., and Rogers, B. "Herpes Simplex Virus, Varicella-Zoster Virus, Human Herpesvirus 6, and Human Herpesvirus 7." In *Diagnostic Microbiology of the Immunocompromised Host*, edited by Randall T. Hayden, Karen C. Carroll, Yi-Wei Tang, and Donna M. Wolk, 113–128. Washington, D.C.: ASM Press, 2009.

Riek, R. and Eisenberg, D.S. "The Activities of Amyloids from a Structural Perspective." *Nature* 539, no. 7628 (November 2016): 227–35.

Robbins, John. *Healthy at 100: The Scientifically Proven Secrets of the World's Healthiest and Longest-Lived Peoples*. New York: Random House, 2006. 91. Print.

Roberts, C. G., Gurisik, E., Biden, T. J., Sutherland, R. L., and Butt, A. J. "Synergistic Cytotoxicity Between Tamoxifen and the Plant Toxin Persin in Human Breast Cancer Cells Is Dependent on Bim Expression and Mediated by Modulation of Ceramide Metabolism." *Molecular Cancer Therapeutics* 6, no. 10 (October 2007): 27772785.

Rochfort, S. and Panozzo, J. "Phytochemicals for Health, the Role of Pulses." Journal of Agricultural and Food Chemistry 55, no. 20 (October 2007): 7981–7994, PMID: 17784726.

Rodriguez-Amaya, D. B. "Latin American Food Sources of Carotenoids." *Archivos Latinoamericanos de Nutricion* 49, 3 (1999): S74–S84.

Roger, H. E. and Kim, Y. S. "Digestion and Absorption of Dietary Protein." *Annual Review of Medicine* 41 (February 1990): 133–139.

Rojkovich, B., Nagy, E., Pröhle, T., Poór, G., and Gergely, P. "Urinary Excretion of Thiol Compounds in Patients with Rheumatoid Arthritis." *Clinical and Diagnostic Laboratory Immunology* 66, no. 5 (1999): 683–685.

Roxas, M. "The Role of Enzyme Supplementation in Digestive Disorders." *Alternative Medicine Review* 13, no. 4 (December 2008): 307–314, PMID: 19152478.

Roy, S. K., Srivastava, R. K., and Shankar, S. "Inhibition of PI3K/AKT and MAPK/ERK Pathways Causes Activation of FOXO Transcription Factor, Leading to Cell Cycle Arrest and Apoptosis in Pancreatic Cancer." *Journal of Molecular Signaling* 5, no. 1 (July 2010): 10, PMID: 20642839.

Ruano-Ravina, A., Barros-Dios, J. M., Figueiras, A., and Brañas-Tato, P. "Correspondence re Yuan JM et al, Prediagnostic Levels of Serum Beta-Cryptoxanthin and Retinol Predict Smoking-Related Lung Cancer Risk in Shanghai, China." *Cancer Epidemiology, Biomarkers & Prevention: A Publication of the American Association for* Cancer Research, *cosponsored by the American Society of Preventive Oncology* 10, no. 4 (2001): 767–773.

Rustom, I.Y. "Aflatoxin in Food and Feed: Occurrence, Legislation and Inactivation by Physical Methods." *Food Chemistry* 59, no. 1 (1997): 57–67.

Ryan, E., Aherne, S. A., O'Grady, M. N., McGovern, L., Kerry, J. P., and O'Brien, N. M. "Bioactivity of Herb-Enriched Beef Patties." Journal of Medicinal Food 12, no. 4 (August 2009): 893–901, PMID: 19735192.

Samsel, A. and Seneff, S. "Glyphosate, Pathways to Modern Diseases II: Celiac Sprue and Gluten Intolerance." *Interdisciplinary Toxicology* 6, no. 4 (2013): 159–184. http://doi.org/10.2478/intox-2013-0026.

Sandhu, A. K. and Gu, L. "Antioxidant Capacity, Phenolic Content, and Profiling of Phenolic Compounds in the Seeds, Skin, and Pulp of *Vitis Rotundifolia* (Muscadine Grapes) as Determined by HPLC-DAD-ESI-MS(N)." Journal of Agricultural and Food Chemistry 58, no. 8 (April 2010): 4681–4692, PMID: 20334341.

Saracino, M. A. and Raggi, M. A. "Analysis of Soy Isoflavone Plasma Levels Using HPLC with Coulometric Detection in Postmenopausal Women." *Journal of Pharmaceutical and Biomedical Analysis* 53, no. 3 (November 2010): 682–687, PMID: 20580512.

Sari, A., Sobocanec, S., Balog, T., Kusi, B., Sverko, V., Dragovi-Uzelac, V., Levaj, B., Cosi, Z., Macak Safranko, Z., and Marotti, T. "Improved Antioxidant and Anti-Inflammatory Potential in Mice Consuming Sour Cherry Juice (*Prunus Cerasus Cv. Maraska*)." *Plant Foods for Human Nutrition* 64, no. 4 (December 2009): 231–237, PMID: 19763832.

Satia, J. A., Tseng, M., Galenko, J. A., Martin, C., and Sandler, R. S. "Associations of Micronutrients with Colon Cancer Risk in African Americans and Whites: Results from the North Carolina Colon Cancer Study." *Cancer Epidemiology and Prevention Biomarkers* 12, no. 8 (2003): 747–754. PMID: 15066939.

Schirrmacher, G., Skurk, T., Hauner, H., and Grassmann, J. "Effect of *Spinacia Oleraceae L.* and *Perilla Frutescens L.* on Antioxidants and Lipid Peroxidation in an Intervention Study in

Healthy Individuals." *Plant Foods for Human Nutrition* 65, no. 1 (March 2010): 71–76, PMID: 20052549.

Schuld, A., Birkmann, S., Beitinger, P., Haack, M., Kraus, T., Dalal, M. A., Holsboer, F., and Pollmächer, T. "Low Doses of Dexamethasone Affect Immune Parameters in the Absence of Immunological Stimulation." *Experimental and Clinical Endocrinology and Diabetes* 114, no. 6 (June 2006): 322–328, PMID: 16868892.

Seaborn, C. D. and Nielsen, F. H. "Dietary Silicon and Arginine Affect Mineral Element Composition of Rat Femur and Vertebra." *Biological Trace Element Research* 89, no. 3 (December 2002): 239–250.

Seker, M., Gül, M. K., Ipek, M., Toplu, C., and Kaleci, N. "Screening and Comparing Tocopherols in the Rapeseed (*Brassica Napus L.*) and Olive (*Olea Europaea L.*) Varieties Using High-Performance Liquid Chromatography." International Journal of Food Sciences and Nutrition 59, no. 6 (September 2008): 483–490, PMID: 19086241.

Serraclara, A., Hawkins, F., Pérez, C., Domínguez, E., Campillo, J. E., and Torres, M. D. "Hypoglycemic Action of an Oral Fig-Leaf Decoction in Type-I Diabetic Patients." *Diabetes Research and Clinical Practice* 39, no. 1 (January 1998): 19–22, PMID: 9597370.

Shafiee, M., Carbonneau, M. A., d'Huart, J. B., Descomps, B., and Léger, C. L. "Synergistic Antioxidative Properties of Phenolics from Natural Origin Toward Low-Density Lipoproteins Depend on the Oxidation System." Journal of Medicinal Food 5, no. 2 (Summer 2002): 69–78, PMID: 12487753.

Shaikh, N., Leonard, E., and Martin, J. M. "Prevalence of Streptococcal Pharyngitis and Streptococcal Carriage in Children: A Meta-Analysis." *Pediatrics* 126, no. 3 (2010): 557–564.

Sheila, L., Gibson, M., Alex, P., Gardner, W., and Gibson, R. G. "A Clinical Evaluation of a Wheat-Free Diet." Journal of Nutritio*nal and Environmental Medicine* 5, no. 3 (January 1995): 243–253.

Singh, H. B., Srivastava, M., Singh, A. B., and Srivastava, A. K. "Cinnamon Bark Oil, A Potent Fungitoxicant Against Fungi Causing Respiratory Tract Mycoses." *Allergy* 50, no. 12 (December 1995): 995–999.

Singh, I., Sagare, A. P., Coma, M., Perlmutter, D., Gelein, R., Bell, R. D., Deane, R. J., et al. "Low Levels of Copper Disrupt Brain Amyloid-B Homeostasis by Altering Its Production and Clearance." *Proceedings of the National Academy of Sciences in the United States of America* 110, no. 36 (2013):14771–6.

Siri-Tarino, P. W., Sun, Q., Hu, F. B., and Krauss, R. M. "Saturated Fatty Acids and Risk of Coronary Heart Disease: Modulation by Replacement Nutrients." *Current Atherosclerosis Reports* 12, no. 6 (August 2010): 384–390, PMID: 20711693.

Smith, K. L. and Guentzel, J. L. "Mercury Concentrations and Omega-3 Fatty Acids in Fish and Shrimp: Preferential Consumption for Maximum Health Benefits." *Marine Pollution Bulletin* 60, no. 9 (July 2010): 1615–1618, PMID: 20633905.

Soylu, E. M., Kurt, S. and Soylu, S. "In Vitro and In Vivo Antifungal Activities of the Essential Oils of Various Plants Against Tomato Grey Mould Disease Agent *Botrytis Cinerea*." International Journal of Food Microbiology 143, no. 3 (August 2010): 183–189, PMID: 20826038.

Srivastava, J. K., Pandey, M., and Gupta, S. "Chamomile, a Novel and Selective COX-2 Inhibitor with Anti-Inflammatory Activity." Life Sciences 85, no. 19-20 (November 2009): 663–669, PMID: 19788894.

Srivastava, R. M., Singh, S., Dubey, S. K., Misra, K., and Khar, A. "Immunomodulatory and Therapeutic Activity of Curcumin." *International Immunopharmacology* 11, no. 3 (September 2011): 331–341, PMID: 20828642.

St. Angelo, A. J. and Ory, R. L. "Effect of Lipoperoxides on Protein in Raw and Processed Peanuts." *LWT-Food Science and Technolology* 4, no. 1 (1975): 26–33.

Stangl, G. I., Schwarz, F. J., Müller, H., and Kirchgessner, M. "Evaluation of the Cobalt Requirement of Beef Cattle Based on Vitamin B12, Folate, Homocysteine and Methylmalonic Acid." The British Journal of Nutrition 84, no. 5 (November 2000): 645–653, PMID: 11177177.

Steinbrecher, A. and Linseisen, J. "Dietary Intake of Individual Glucosinolates in Participants of the EPIC-Heidelberg Cohort Study." *Annals of Nutrition and Metabolism* 54, no. 2 (2009): 87–96.

Strasfeld, L., Romanzi, L., Seder, R. H., and Berardi, V. P. "False-Positive Serological Test Results for Lyme Disease in a Patient with Acute Herpes Simplex Virus Type 2 Infection." *Clinical Infectious Diseases* 15 (December 2005): 1826–1827.

Suganthy, N., Devi, K. P., Nabavi, S. F., Braidy, N., and Nabavi, S. M. "Bioactive Effects of Quercetin in the Central Nervous System: Focusing on the Mechanisms of Actions." *Biomedicine & Pharmacotherapy* 31, no. 84 (December 2016): 892–908.

"Sugar Intake Hit All-Time High in 1999." Center for Science in the Public Interest. Accessed September 26, 2010. http://www.cspinet.org/new/sugar_limit.html.

Sun-Edelstein, C. and Mauskop, A. "Foods and Supplements in the Management of Migraine Headaches." *The Clinical Journal of Pain* 25, no. 5 (June 2009): 446–452, PMID: 19454881.

"Sustainable Agriculture: Definitions and Terms." National Agricultural Library. Accessed Sept 27, 2010. http://www.nal.usda.gov/afsic/pubs/terms/srb9902.shtml.

Tapp, L. and Sylvain, D. "Skin and Respiratory Symptoms in Peanut Inspectors with Peanut Dust and Endotoxin Exposure." *Journal of Occupational and Environmental Hygiene* 10, no. 2 (2013): D19-24.

"The PH Equation & Health." Biomedx: Science and Logic for Health. Accessed September 26, 2010. http://biomedx.com/microscopes/rrintro/rr4.html.

Toda, T., Uesugi, T., Hirai, K., Nukaya, H., Tsuji, K., and Ishida, H. "New 6-O-Acyl Isoflavone Glycosides from Soybeans Fermented with *Bacillus Subtilis (Natto)*. I. 6-O-Succinylated Isoflavone Glycosides and Their Preventive Effects on Bone Loss in Ovariectomized Rats Fed a Calcium-Deficient Diet." Biological and Pharmaceutical Bulletin 22, no. 11 (November 1999): 1193–1201.

Tojo, K., Tokuda, T., Hoshii, Y., Fu, X., Higuchi, K., Matsui, T., Kametani, F. and Ikeda, S. "Unexpectedly High Incidence of Visceral AA-Amyloidosis in Slaughtered Cattle in Japan." *Amyloid* 12, no. 2 (2005): 103–108.

Torpey, J. M., Lynm, C., and Glass, R. "The Metabolic Syndrome." *JAMA* 295, no. 7 (February 2006): 850. doi:10.1001/jama.295.7.850.

"Top 20 Antioxidant-Rich Foods." NHL Ministries. Accessed September 23, 2010. http://blpublications.com/html/top20antioxidant.html.

Trentham-Dietz, A. "Total Xenoestrogen Body Burden in Relation to Mammographic Density, a Marker of Breast Cancer Risk." *The Government Reports Announcements & Index (GRA&I)* 23 (2008). Accessed January 26, 2018. http://www.dtic.mil/dtic/tr/fulltext/u2/a501848.pdf.

Ulmius, M., Johansson and A., and Onning, G. "The Influence of Dietary Fibre Source and Gender on the Postprandial Glucose and Lipid Response in Healthy Subjects." *European Journal of Nutrition* 48, no. 7 (October 2009): 395–402, PMID: 19415409.

Uma Devi, P. "Radioprotective, Anticarcinogenic and Antioxidant Properties of the Indian Holy Basil, *Ocimum santum (Tulasi)*." *Indian Journal of Experimental Biology* 39, no. 3 (2001): 185–190.

"Understanding Your Energy Body." Kahunka Health and Fitness. Accessed September 27, 2010. http://kahunka.com/original-articles/understanding-your-energy-body.

"USDA Science Unlocks the Genetic Secrets of the Soybean." USDA Blog. Accessed September 27, 2010. http://blogs.usda.gov/tag/soybean/.

United States Department of Agriculture (USDA). "Classification for Kingdom Plantae Down to Family Fabaceae." Accessed April 16, 2005. http://www.plants.usda.gov/java/ClassificationServlet?source=profile&symbol=Fabaceae&display=63.

United States Department of Agriculture (USDA). "Inside the Pyramid." MyPyramid.gov. Accessed July 23, 2014. http://www.mypyramid.gov/pyramid/index.html.

United States Department of Agriculture (USDA), Economic Research Service (ERS). *Adoption of Genetically Engineered Crops in the U.S.: Extent of Adoption.* Accessed July 3, 2012. Distributed by USDA ERS. https://www.ers.usda.gov/data-products/adoption-of-genetically-engineered-crops-in-the-us.aspx.

United States Department of Health and Human Services (HHS). "U.S. Food and Drug Administration (FDA) Requires Boxed Warning and Risk Mitigation Strategy for Metoclopramide-Containing Drugs: Agency Warns against Chronic Use of These Products to Treat Gastrointestinal Disorders." Fda.gov. Accessed February 26, 2009. https://www.fiercebiotech.com/biotech/fda-requires-boxed-warning-and-risk-mitigation-strategy-for-metoclopramide-containing-drugs.

United States Environmental Protection Agency (EPA). "What You Need to Know about Mercury in Fish and Shellfish Outreach & Communication—US EPA." Last modified September 27, 2010. http://water.epa.gov/scitech/swguidance/fishshellfish/outreach/advice_index.cfm.

Valentine, Judith. "The Dangers of Soft Drinks—America." Global Healing Center Health Products & Information. Accessed September 26, 2010. http://www.globalhealingcenter.com/soft-drinks-america.html.

Váli, L., Stefanovits-Bányai, E., Szentmihályi, K., Fébel, H., Sárdi, E., Lugasi, A., Kocsis, I., and Blázovics, A. "Liver-Protecting Effects of Table Beet (*Beta Vulgaris Var. Rubra*) During Ischemia-Reperfusion." *Nutrition* 23, no. 2 (February 2007): 172–178, PMID: 17234508.

van Breemen, R. B., Tao, Y., and Li, W. "Cyclooxygenase-2 Inhibitors in Ginger (*Zingiber Officinale*)." *Fitoterapia* 82, no. 1 (September 2010): 38–43, PMID: 20837112.

van Poppel, G., Verhoeven, D. T., Verhagen, H., and Goldbohm, R. A. "Brassica Vegetables and Cancer Preventon. Epidemiology and Mechanisms." *Advances in Experimental Medicine and Biology* 472 (1999): 159–168.

"Vegetable." Encyclopedia Britannica. Accessed August 13, 2008. http://www.britannica.com/EBchecked/topic/624564/vegetable.

Verhoven, D. T., Goldbom, R. A., van Poppel, G., Verhagen, H. and van den Brandt, P.A. "Epidemiological Studies on Brassica Vegetables and Cancer Risk." *Cancer Epidemiology Biomarkers and Prevention* 5, no. 9 (1996): 773–748.

Vibin, M., Siva-Priya, S. G., Rooban, B., Sasikala, V., Sahasranamam, V., and Abraham, A. "Broccoli Regulates Protein Alterations and Cataractogenesis in Selenite Models." *Current Eye Research* 35, no. 2 (February 2010): 99–107, PMID: 20136419.

Visentín, A. N., Drago, S. R., Osella, C. A., de la Torre, M. A., Sánchez, H. D., and González, R. J. "Effect of the Addition of Soy Flour and Whey Protein Concentrate on Bread Quality and Mineral Dialyzability." *Archivos Latinoamericanos de Nutricion* 59, no. 3 (September 2009): 325–331, PMID: 19886519.

Vogel, J. T., Tieman, D. M., Sims, C. A., Odabasi, A. Z., Clark, D. G., and Klee, H. J. "Carotenoid Content Impacts Flavor Acceptability in Tomato (*Solanum Lycopersicum*)." *Journal of Science and Food Agriculture* 90, no. 13 (July 2010): 2233–2240, PMID: 20661902.

Voorrips, L. E., Goldbohm, R. A., van Poppel, G., Sturmans, F., Hermus, R. J., and van den Brandt, P. A. "Vegetable and Fruit Consumption and Risks of Colon and Rectal Cancer in a Prospective Cohort Study: The Netherlands Cohort Study on Diet and Cancer." *American Journal of Epidemiology* 152, no. 11 (December 2000): 1081–1092, PMID: 11117618.

Vrinda, B. and Uma Devi, P. "Radiation Protection of Human Lymphocyte Chromosomes in vitro by Orientin and Vicenin." *Mutation Research* 498, no. 1–2 (2001): 39–46.

Waliszewski, K. N. and Blasco, G. "Nutraceutical Properties of Lycopene." *Salud Publica de Mexico* 52, no. 3 (May-June 2010): 254–265.

Walters, M. and Sperandio, V. "Autoinducer 3 and Epinephrine Signaling in the Kinetics of Locus of Enterocyte Effacement Gene Expression in Enterohemorrhagic Escherichia Coli." *Infection and Immunity* 74, no. 10 (2006): 5445–5455, http://doi.org/10.1128/IAI.00099-06.

Waring, R.H. and Emery, P. "Management of Early Inflammatory Arthritis. Genetic Factors Predicting Persistent Disease: The Role of Defective Enzyme Systems." *Bailliere's Clinical Rheumatology* 6, no. 2 (June 1992): 337–50.

Washington State University. "Commercial Organic Farms Have Better Fruit and Soil, Lower Environmental Impact, Study Finds." *Science Daily: News & Articles in Science, Health, Environment & Technology,* September 2, 2010. http://www.sciencedaily.com/releases/2010/09/100901171553.htm.

Wender, E. H. "The Food Additive-Free Diet in the Treatment of Behavior Disorders: A Review." *Journal of Developmental and Behavioral Pediatrics* 7, no. 1 (February 1986): 35–42, PMID: 3949989.

Whelton, P. K. and He, J. "Potassium in Preventing and Treating High Blood Pressure." *Seminars in Nephrology* 19, no. 5 (1999): 494–499.

White, Donald, ed. *Compendium of Corn Diseases (Third Issue).* St Paul, MN: The American Phytopathological Society, 1999.

Wiboonpun, N., Phuwapraisiriasan, P., and Tippyang, S. "Identification of Antioxidant Compound from *Asparagus Racemosus.*" *Phytotherapy Research* 18, no. 9 (2004): 771–773.

Wilkinson, A. S., Monteith, G. R., Shaw P. N., Lin, C. N., Gidley, M. J., and Roberts-Thomson, S. J. "Effects of the Mango Components Mangiferin and Quercetin and the Putative Mangiferin Metabolite Norathyriol on the Transactivation of Peroxisome Proliferator-Acti Vated Receptor Isoforms." Journal of Agricultural and Food Chemistry 56, no. 9 (May 2008): 3037–3042.

Williams, C. D., Satia, J. A., Adair, L. S., Stevens, J., Galanko, J., Keku, T. O., and Sandler, R. S. "Antioxidant and DNA Methylation-Related Nutrients and Risk of Distal Colorectal Cancer." Cancer Causes *Control* 21, no. 8 (August 2010): 1171–1181, PMID: 20352485.

Williams, S. M., Venn, B. J., Perry, T., Brown, R., Wallace, A., Mann, J. I., and Green, T. J. "Another Approach to Estimating the Reliability of Glycaemic Index." *British* Journal of Nutrition 100, no. 2 (2008): 364–372. PMID: 18186950.

Wilson, T. A., Nicolosi, R. J., Woolfrey, B., and Kritchevsky, D. "Rice Bran Oil and Oryzanol Reduce Plasma Lipid and Lipoprotein Cholesterol Concentrations and Aortic Cholesterol Ester Accumulation to a Greater Extent than Ferulic Acid in Hypercholesterolemic Hamsters." *The* Journal of Nutrition*al Biochemistry* 18, no. 2 (February 2007): 105–112, PMID: 16713234.

Woelfle, J., Wilske, B., Haverkamp, F., and Bialek, R. "False-Positive Serological Tests for Lyme Disease in Facial Palsy and Varicella Zoster Meningo-Encephalitis." *European Journal of Pediatrics* 157, no. 11 (1998): 953–4.

Wolkowitz O. M., Reus V. I., and Mellon S. H. "Of Sound Mind and Body: Depression, Disease, and Accelerated Aging." *Dialogues in Clinical Neuroscience* 13, no. 1 (2011): 25–39.

Wood, J. D., Enser, M., Fisher, A. V., Nute, G. R., Sheard, P. R., Richardson, R. I., and Whittington, F. M. "Fat Deposition, Fatty Acid Composition and Meat Quality: A Review." *Meat Science* 78, no. 4 (2008): 343–358.

Xu, W. S., Chan, A. C., Lee, J. M., Liang, R. H., Ho, F. C., and Srivastava, G. "Epstein-Barr Virus Infection and Its Gene Expression in Gastric Lymphoma of Mucosa-Associated Lymphoid Tissue." *Journal of Medical Virology* 56, no. 4 (December 1998): 342–50.

Yamada, M., Kotani, Y., Nakamura, K., Kobayashi, Y., Horiuchi, N., Doi, T., Suzuki, S., Sato, N., Kanno, T., and Matsui, T. "Immunohistochemical Distribution of Amyloid Deposits in 25 Cows Diagnosed with Systemic AA Amyloidosis." *Journal of Veterinary Medical Science* 68, no. 7 (2006): 725–729.

Yang, D., Pornpattananangkul, D., Nakatsuji, T., Chan, M., Carson, D., Huang, C. M., and Zhang, L. "The Antimicrobial Activity of Liposomal Lauric Acids Against *Propionibacterium Acnes*." *Biomaterials* 30, no. 30 (October 2009): 6035–6040, PMID: 19665786; PMCID: PMC2735618.

Yang, Y., Zhou, L., Gu, Y., Zhang, Y., Tang, J., Li, F., Shang, W., Jiang, B., Yue, X., and Chen, M. "Dietary Chickpeas Reverse Visceral Adiposity, Dyslipidaemia and Insulin Resistance in Rats Induced by a Chronic High-Fat Diet." *British* Journal of Nutrition 98, no. 4 (October 2007): 720-776, PMID: 17666145.

Young, R. O. and Redford, S. *The PH Miracle: Balance Your Diet, Reclaim Your Health*. New York: Wellness Central, 2003. 71–73. Print.

Zakpaa, H. D., Mak-Mensah, E. E., and Adubofour, J. "Production and Characterization of Flour Produced from Ripe "Apem" Plantain (*Musa Sapientum L. Var. Paradisiacal*; French Horn) Grown in Ghana." *Journal of Agricultural Biotechnology and Sustainable Development* 2, no. 6 (June 2010): 92–99.

Zeng, H. and Botnen, J. H. "Selenium is Critical for Cancer-Signaling Gene Expression but Not Cell Proliferation in Human Colon Caco-2 Cells." *Biofactors* 31, no. 3-4 (2007): 155–164.

Zhou, L., Zhang, Y., Gapter, L. A., Ling, H., Agarwal, R., and Ng, K. Y. "Cytotoxic and Anti-Oxidant Activities of Lanostane-Type Triterpenes Isolated from *Poria Cocos*." *Chemical and Pharmaceutical Bulletin (Tokyo)* 56, no. 10 (October 2008): 1459–1462, PMID: 18827390.

Zhou, Y. J., Zhang, S. P., Liu, C. W., and Cai, Y. Q. "The Protection of Selenium on ROS Mediated-Apoptosis by Mitochondria Dysfunction in Cadmium-Induced LLC-PK (1) Cells." *Toxicology In Vitro* 23, no. 2 (March 2009): 288–294.

Zhu, B. T., Loder, D. P., Cai, M. X., Ho, C. T., Huang, M. T., and Conney, A. H. "Dietary Administration of an Extract from Rosemary Leaves Enhances the Liver Microsomal Metabolism of Endogenous Estrogens and Decreases Their Uterotropic Action in CD-1 Mice." *Carcinogenesis* 19, no. 10 (October 1998): 1821–1827.

Zhuo, J. M., Portugal, G. S., Kruger, W. D., Wang, H., Gould, T. J., and Pratico, D. "Diet-Induced Hyperhomocysteinemia Increases Amyloid-Formation and Deposition in a Mouse Model of Alzheimer's Disease." Current Alzheimer Research 7, no. 2 (March 2010): 140–149.

ADDITIONAL RESOURCES

1. **Guide to pesticides in produce**

   EWG *Dirty Dozen* app or visit *www.ewg.org*

---

2. **Avoiding GMO foods**

   Non-GMO Project app or
   visit *www.nongmoproject.org*

---

3. **Avoiding toxic cleaning products**

   www.ewg.org/guides/cleaners

---

4. **Choosing cleaner food**

   EWG *Healthy Living* app or visit *www.ewg.org*

---

5. **Choosing clean personal care products**

   EWG *Healthy Living* app or visit *www.ewg.org*

---

6. **Guide to clean seafood**

   www.ewg.org/research/ewgs-good-seafood-guide
   www.nrdc.org/stories/smart-seafood-buying-guide

---

7. **Advice on having a healthy home**

   www.ewg.org/healthyhomeguide

---

8. **Stress management & relaxation resources**

   www.HeartMath.com
   Smartphone apps, for example:
   Calm, *Headspace*, *Insight Timer*

---

9. Wild meats online

www.DArtagnan.com
www.SteaksAndGame.com
www.Cabelas.com
www.FossilFarms.com
www.VermontQuail.com
www.PheasantForDinner.com
www.PrairieHarvest.com
www.Squab.com
www.ManchesterFarms.com
www.NebraskaBison.com
www.jhBuffaloMeat.com
www.AllenBrothers.com

---

10. Clean fish and seafood online

www.VitalChoice.com

---

11. Wildatarian™ pantry basics

www.ThriveMarket.com

---

12. Wildatarian HealAndSeal™ Program

www.TeriCochrane.com

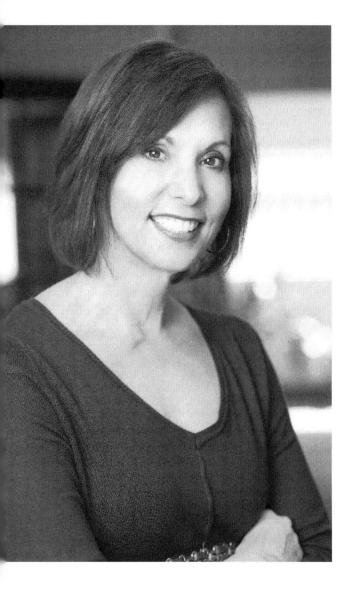

ABOUT THE AUTHOR

Teri Cochrane is an integrative practitioner and thought leader in nutritional counseling. She earned a Bachelor of Science degree from the University of Florida, and she is a graduate of the Huntington College of Health Sciences and the National Leadership Institute. She also has extensive certifications and experience in holistic medicinal practices, such as healing touch, craniosacral therapy, meditation techniques, certified coaching, and herbology. She has developed her own methodology, "The Cochrane Method," which integrates a multi-level nutritional approach, including observation and listening, to develop a bio-individualized plan for her clients. She is a writer and speaker and maintains a nationally read blog and radio presence.

Teri is currently in private practice in the Washington, D.C. Metropolitan area, where she specializes in complex health conditions. She also specializes in elite athletic performance. She serves as a nutritional counselor to ballerinas and Olympic hopefuls, including one of the most promising young swimmers in the country.

Teri's approach and voice have been extended to the national and international audience through media appearances, which include the medical lifestyle show *Ask Dr. Nandi* with Dr. Partha Nandi and the docuseries *The Thyroid Secret* with Izabella Wentz. Teri is a frequent guest on blog radio, including *Thyroid Nation, Unlimited Realities,* and *Life Mastery Radio.* She regularly lectures at the Washington School of Ballet. She has lectured at several major hospitals in Virginia, including INOVA, Virginia Hospital Center, and Fair Oaks Hospital. She also has been featured in publications including *The Washington Post.*